NATIONAL ACADEMIES *Sciences Engineering Medicine*

NATIONAL ACADEMIES PRESS
Washington, DC

Innovation in Electronic Health Records for Oncology Care, Research, and Surveillance

Erin Balogh, Francis Amankwah, Theresa Wizemann, and Sharyl Nass, *Rapporteurs*

National Cancer Policy Forum

Board on Health Care Services

Health and Medicine Division

Computer Science and Telecommunications Board

Division on Engineering and Physical Sciences

Proceedings of a Workshop

THE NATIONAL ACADEMIES PRESS 500 Fifth Street, NW Washington, DC 20001

This activity was supported by Contract No. 75D30121D11240 (Task Order No. 75D30121F00002) and Contract No. HHSN263201800029I (Task Order No. HHSN26300008) with the Centers for Disease Control and Prevention and the National Cancer Institute/National Institutes of Health, respectively, and by the American Association for Cancer Research, American Cancer Society, American College of Radiology, American Society of Clinical Oncology, Association of American Cancer Institutes, Association of Community Cancer Centers, Bristol Myers Squibb, Cancer Support Community, Flatiron Health, Merck & Co., Inc., National Comprehensive Cancer Network, National Patient Advocate Foundation, Novartis Oncology, Oncology Nursing Society, Partners in Health, Pfizer Inc., Sanofi, and Society for Immunotherapy of Cancer. Any opinions, findings, conclusions, or recommendations expressed in this publication do not necessarily reflect the views of any organization or agency that provided support for the project.

International Standard Book Number-13: 978-0-309-69387-5
International Standard Book Number-10: 0-309-69387-X
Digital Object Identifier: https://doi.org/10.17226/26720

This publication is available from the National Academies Press, 500 Fifth Street, NW, Keck 360, Washington, DC 20001; (800) 624-6242 or (202) 334-3313; http://www.nap.edu.

Copyright 2023 by the National Academy of Sciences. National Academies of Sciences, Engineering, and Medicine and National Academies Press and the graphical logos for each are all trademarks of the National Academies of Sciences. All rights reserved.

Suggested citation: National Academies of Sciences, Engineering, and Medicine. 2023. *Innovation in electronic health records for oncology care, research, and surveillance: Proceedings of a workshop.* Washington, DC: The National Academies Press. https://doi.org/10.17226/26720.

The **National Academy of Sciences** was established in 1863 by an Act of Congress, signed by President Lincoln, as a private, nongovernmental institution to advise the nation on issues related to science and technology. Members are elected by their peers for outstanding contributions to research. Dr. Marcia McNutt is president.

The **National Academy of Engineering** was established in 1964 under the charter of the National Academy of Sciences to bring the practices of engineering to advising the nation. Members are elected by their peers for extraordinary contributions to engineering. Dr. John L. Anderson is president.

The **National Academy of Medicine** (formerly the Institute of Medicine) was established in 1970 under the charter of the National Academy of Sciences to advise the nation on medical and health issues. Members are elected by their peers for distinguished contributions to medicine and health. Dr. Victor J. Dzau is president.

The three Academies work together as the **National Academies of Sciences, Engineering, and Medicine** to provide independent, objective analysis and advice to the nation and conduct other activities to solve complex problems and inform public policy decisions. The National Academies also encourage education and research, recognize outstanding contributions to knowledge, and increase public understanding in matters of science, engineering, and medicine.

Learn more about the National Academies of Sciences, Engineering, and Medicine at **www.nationalacademies.org**.

Consensus Study Reports published by the National Academies of Sciences, Engineering, and Medicine document the evidence-based consensus on the study's statement of task by an authoring committee of experts. Reports typically include findings, conclusions, and recommendations based on information gathered by the committee and the committee's deliberations. Each report has been subjected to a rigorous and independent peer-review process and it represents the position of the National Academies on the statement of task.

Proceedings published by the National Academies of Sciences, Engineering, and Medicine chronicle the presentations and discussions at a workshop, symposium, or other event convened by the National Academies. The statements and opinions contained in proceedings are those of the participants and are not endorsed by other participants, the planning committee, or the National Academies.

Rapid Expert Consultations published by the National Academies of Sciences, Engineering, and Medicine are authored by subject-matter experts on narrowly focused topics that can be supported by a body of evidence. The discussions contained in rapid expert consultations are considered those of the authors and do not contain policy recommendations. Rapid expert consultations are reviewed by the institution before release.

For information about other products and activities of the National Academies, please visit www.nationalacademies.org/about/whatwedo.

PLANNING COMMITTEE[1]

MIA LEVY (*Co-Chair*), Chief Medical Officer, Foundation Medicine, Inc.
LAWRENCE N. SHULMAN (*Co-Chair*), Professor of Medicine, Deputy Director for Clinical Services, and Director of the Center for Global Cancer Medicine, Abramson Cancer Center, University of Pennsylvania
ROBERT W. CARLSON, Chief Executive Officer, National Comprehensive Cancer Network
NICOLE F. DOWLING, Associate Director for Science, Division of Cancer Prevention and Control, National Center for Chronic Disease Prevention and Health Promotion, Centers for Disease Control and Prevention
MIMI HUIZINGA, Senior Vice President and Head of Medical Affairs, ImmunoGen, Inc.
BRADLEY MALIN, Accenture Professor of Biomedical Informatics, Biostatistics, and Computer Science and Vice Chair for Research Affairs, Department of Biomedical Informatics, Vanderbilt University Medical Center
ALEXANDER MELAMED, Assistant Professor, Department of Obstetrics and Gynecology, Columbia University Medical Center, New York Presbyterian Hospital
NEAL MEROPOL, Vice President, Research Oncology, Flatiron Health; and Adjunct Professor, Case Comprehensive Cancer Center
ETTA D. PISANO, Senior Director for Research Development, Center for Research and Innovation, American College of Radiology; and Vice Chair for Research, Department of Radiology, Beth Israel Deaconess Medical Center
JULIE SCHNEIDER, Associate Director, Research Strategy and Partnership, Oncology Center of Excellence, Food and Drug Administration
ROBERT A. WINN, Director, Massey Cancer Center, Senior Associate Dean for Cancer Innovation, Professor of Pulmonary Disease and Critical Care Medicine, and Lipman Chair in Oncology, School of Medicine, Virginia Commonwealth University; and President-Elect, Association of American Cancer Institutes

---

[1] The National Academies of Sciences, Engineering, and Medicine's planning committees are solely responsible for organizing the workshop, identifying topics, and choosing speakers. The responsibility for the published Proceedings of a Workshop rests with the workshop rapporteurs and the institution.

ROBIN YABROFF, Scientific Vice President, Health Services Research, American Cancer Society

Project Staff

FRANCIS AMANKWAH, Program Officer
RACHEL AUSTIN, Senior Program Assistant (*until June 2022*)
LORI BENJAMIN BRENIG, Research Associate
ANNALEE GONZALES, Administrative Assistant (*until May 2022*)
ARZOO TAYYEB, Finance Business Partner
ERIN BALOGH, Co-Director, National Cancer Policy Forum
SHARYL J. NASS, Co-Director, National Cancer Policy Forum; and Senior Director, Board on Health Care Services

NATIONAL CANCER POLICY FORUM[1]

EDWARD J. BENZ, JR. (*Chair*), President and Chief Executive Officer, Emeritus, Dana-Farber Cancer Institute; and Richard and Susan Smith Distinguished Professor of Medicine, Genetics, and Pediatrics, Harvard Medical School
PETER C. ADAMSON, Global Head, Oncology Development and Pediatric Innovation, Sanofi
GARNET L. ANDERSON, Senior Vice President and Director, Public Health Sciences Division, Fred Hutchinson Cancer Center; Affiliate Professor, Department of Biostatistics, University of Washington; and Principal Investigator, Women's Health Initiative Clinical Coordinating Center
KAREN BASEN-ENGQUIST, Annie Laurie Howard Research Distinguished Professor, Director of the Center for Energy Balance in Cancer Prevention and Survivorship, and Professor of Behavioral Science, The University of Texas MD Anderson Cancer Center
SMITA BHATIA, Director, Institute for Cancer Outcomes and Survivorship, Gay and Bew White Endowed Chair in Pediatric Oncology, and Professor and Vice Chair of Outcomes for Pediatrics, School of Medicine, The University of Alabama at Birmingham
CHRIS BOSHOFF, Chief Development Officer, Oncology and Rare Disease, Global Product Development, Pfizer Inc.
CATHY J. BRADLEY, David F. and Margaret Turley Grohne Endowed Chair for Cancer Prevention and Control Research, Professor and Associate Dean for Research, Colorado School of Public Health, and Bunn Chair of Cancer Research and Deputy Director, University of Colorado Cancer Center
OTIS W. BRAWLEY, Bloomberg Distinguished Professor, Department of Epidemiology and Oncology, Bloomberg School of Public Health and Department of Oncology, School of Medicine, Sidney Kimmel Comprehensive Cancer Center, Johns Hopkins University
ROBERT W. CARLSON, Chief Executive Officer, National Comprehensive Cancer Network

---

[1] The National Academies of Sciences, Engineering, and Medicine's forums and roundtables do not issue, review, or approve individual documents. The responsibility for the published Proceedings of a Workshop rests with the workshop rapporteurs and the institution.

CHRISTINA CHAPMAN, Assistant Professor of Radiation Oncology, Baylor College of Medicine
GWEN DARIEN, Executive Vice President, Patient Advocacy and Engagement, National Patient Advocate Foundation
NANCY E. DAVIDSON, Executive Vice President for Clinical Affairs, Senior Vice President and Professor, Clinical Research Division, and Raisbeck Endowed Chair for Collaborative Cancer Research, Fred Hutchinson Cancer Center; Professor and Head, Division of Medical Oncology, Department of Medicine, University of Washington
JAMES H. DOROSHOW, Director, Division of Cancer Treatment and Diagnosis, Deputy Director for Clinical and Translational Research, and Head of the Oxidative Signaling and Molecular Therapeutics Group, National Cancer Institute of the National Institutes of Health
NICOLE F. DOWLING, Associate Director for Science, Division of Cancer Prevention and Control, National Center for Chronic Disease Prevention and Health Promotion, Centers for Disease Control and Prevention
SCOT W. EBBINGHAUS, Vice President and Therapeutic Area Head, Oncology Clinical Research, Merck Research Laboratories
KOJO S. J. ELENITOBA-JOHNSON, Inaugural Chair of the Department of Pathology and Laboratory Medicine, Memorial Sloan Kettering Cancer Center
STANTON L. GERSON, Dean and Senior Vice President, Medical Affairs, Case Western Reserve University School of Medicine; Acting Director, Case Comprehensive Cancer Center; Asa & Patricia Shiverick–Jane B. Shiverick (Tripp) Professor of Hematological Oncology and Distinguished University Professor and Director, National Center for Regenerative Medicine, Case Western Reserve University
JULIE R. GRALOW, Chief Medical Officer and Executive Vice Present, American Society of Clinical Oncology
ROY S. HERBST, Ensign Professor of Medicine, Professor of Pharmacology, Chief of Medical Oncology, and Associate Director for Translational Research, Yale Cancer Center and Yale School of Medicine
HEDVIG HRICAK, Carroll and Milton Petrie Chair, Department of Radiology, Memorial Sloan Kettering Cancer Center; Professor of Radiology, Weill Medical College, Cornell University; and Professor, Gerstner Sloan-Kettering Graduate School of Biomedical Sciences

CHANITA HUGHES-HALBERT, Vice Chair for Research, Professor in the Department of Preventive Medicine, and Associate Director for Cancer Equity, Norris Comprehensive Cancer Center, Keck School of Medicine, University of Southern California

ROY A. JENSEN, Vice Chancellor and Director, The University of Kansas Cancer Center, William R. Jewell, M.D. Distinguished Kansas Masonic Professor of Cancer Research, Director, Kansas Masonic Cancer Research Institute, and Professor of Pathology and Laboratory Medicine, Cancer Biology, Anatomy and Cell Biology, University of Kansas Medical Center, and Past President, Association of American Cancer Institutes

RANDY A. JONES, Professor and Associate Dean for Partner Development and Engagement, University of Virginia School of Nursing; and Assistant Director, Community Outreach and Engagement, Emily Couric Clinical Cancer Center, University of Virginia

BETH Y. KARLAN, Nancy Marks Endowed Chair in Women's Health Research, Vice Chair and Professor, Department of Obstetrics and Gynecology, Director, Cancer Population Genetics, Jonsson Comprehensive Cancer Center, University of California, Los Angeles

SAMIR N. KHLEIF, Director, Jeannie and Tony Loop Immuno-Oncology Lab; Biomedical Scholar and Professor of Oncology, Georgetown Lombardi Comprehensive Cancer Center, Georgetown University Medical Center; and Member, Society for Immunotherapy of Cancer

MIA LEVY, Chief Medical Officer, Foundation Medicine, Inc.

SCOTT M. LIPPMAN, Director, Moores Cancer Center and Distinguished Professor of Medicine, Senior Associate Dean, Associate Vice Chancellor for Cancer Research and Care, and Chugai Pharmaceutical Chair in Cancer, University of California, San Diego

LARISSA NEKHLYUDOV, Professor of Medicine, Harvard Medical School; Internist, Brigham and Women's Hospital; and Clinical Director, Internal Medicine for Cancer Survivors, Dana-Farber Cancer Institute

RANDALL A. OYER, Clinical Professor of Medicine, Perelman School of Medicine; Executive Medical Director, Ann B. Barshinger Cancer Institute, Penn Medicine Lancaster General Health; and Past President, Association of Community Cancer Centers

CLEO A. RYALS, Head of Health Equity and Health Disparities Research, Flatiron Health

RICHARD L. SCHILSKY, Principal Investigator, ASCO TAPUR Study; and Professor Emeritus, University of Chicago
JULIE SCHNEIDER, Associate Director, Research Strategy and Partnership, Oncology Center of Excellence, Food and Drug Administration
SUSAN M. SCHNEIDER, Associate Professor Emerita, School of Nursing, Duke University
LAWRENCE N. SHULMAN, Professor of Medicine, Deputy Director for Clinical Services, and Director, Center for Global Cancer Medicine, Abramson Cancer Center, University of Pennsylvania
HEIDI SMITH, Vice President, Center of Operations and Research Excellence, U.S. Clinical Development and Medical Affairs, Oncology, Novartis Pharmaceuticals
LARA STRAWBRIDGE, Director, Division of Ambulatory Payment Models, Patient Care Models Group, Center for Medicare and Medicaid Innovation, Centers for Medicare & Medicaid Services
GEORGE J. WEINER, Director of the Holden Comprehensive Cancer Center at The University of Iowa, C. E. Block Chair of Cancer Research, and Professor of Internal Medicine and Pharmaceutical Science, University of Iowa
ROBERT A. WINN, Director, Massey Cancer Center, Senior Associate Dean for Cancer Innovation, Professor of Pulmonary Disease and Critical Care Medicine, and Lipman Chair in Oncology, School of Medicine, Virginia Commonwealth University; and President-Elect, Association of American Cancer Institutes
ROBIN YABROFF, Scientific Vice President, Health Services Research, American Cancer Society

National Cancer Policy Forum Staff

FRANCIS AMANKWAH, Program Officer
LORI BENJAMIN BRENIG, Research Associate
TORRIE BROWN, Program Coordinator (*from August 2022*)
CHIDINMA CHUKWURAH, Senior Program Assistant (*from August 2022*)
JACARI JENNINGS, Senior Program Assistant (*from July 2022*)
ARZOO TAYYEB, Finance Business Partner
ERIN BALOGH, Co-Director, National Cancer Policy Forum
SHARYL J. NASS, Co-Director, National Cancer Policy Forum; and Senior Director, Board on Health Care Services

Reviewers

This Proceedings of a Workshop was reviewed in draft form by individuals chosen for their diverse perspectives and technical expertise. The purpose of this independent review is to provide candid and critical comments that will assist the National Academies of Sciences, Engineering, and Medicine in making each published report as sound as possible and to ensure that it meets the institutional standards for quality, objectivity, evidence, and responsiveness to the study charge. The review comments and draft manuscript remain confidential to protect the integrity of the deliberative process.

We thank the following individuals for their review of this report:

ETHAN M. BASCH, University of North Carolina
TUFIA C. HADDAD, Mayo Clinic
MATTHEW B. WEINGER, Vanderbilt University Medical Center

Although the reviewers listed above provided many constructive comments and suggestions, they were not asked to endorse the conclusions or recommendations of this report nor did they see the final draft before its release. The review of this report was overseen by **DANIEL R. MASYS,** University of Washington. He was responsible for making certain that an independent examination of this report was carried out in accordance with the standards of the National Academies and that all review comments were carefully considered. Responsibility for the final content rests entirely with the rapporteurs and the National Academies.

Acknowledgments

Support from the many annual sponsors of the National Academies of Sciences, Engineering, and Medicine's National Cancer Policy Forum is crucial to the work of the forum. Federal sponsors include the Centers for Disease Control and Prevention and the National Cancer Institute/National Institutes of Health. Non-federal sponsors include the American Association for Cancer Research, American Cancer Society, American College of Radiology, American Society of Clinical Oncology, Association of American Cancer Institutes, Association of Community Cancer Centers, Bristol Myers Squibb, Cancer Support Community, Flatiron Health, Merck & Co., Inc., National Comprehensive Cancer Network, National Patient Advocate Foundation, Novartis Oncology, Oncology Nursing Society, Partners in Health, Pfizer Inc., Sanofi, and Society for Immunotherapy of Cancer.

The forum wishes to express its gratitude to the expert speakers whose presentations and discussions helped inform efforts to improve the development and use of electronic health records for oncology care, research, and surveillance. The forum also wishes to thank the members of the planning committee for their work in developing an excellent workshop agenda.

Contents

ACRONYMS AND ABBREVIATIONS	xix
PROCEEDINGS OF A WORKSHOP	1
WORKSHOP OVERVIEW	1
OVERVIEW OF THE USE OF EHRs IN ONCOLOGY CARE, RESEARCH, AND SURVEILLANCE	8

    The EHR in Clinical Oncology Practice, 9
    The EHR and the Patient's Relationship with Health
        Care Providers, 11
    The EHR in Quality Improvement and Research, 15

IMPROVING THE PATIENT-FACING ASPECTS OF EHRs	17

    Today's Patient Portal, 17
    The EHR as a Tool for Patient–Clinician Communication, 18
    Integrating Patient-Reported Outcomes into Oncology
        EHR Systems, 20
    Sharing of Patient Data within and among EHR Systems, 22
    Using the EHR to Nudge Evidence-Based Cancer Care, 23
    Next-Generation EHRs, 24

OPTIMIZING THE FUNCTIONALITY AND USABILITY OF EHRs IN ONCOLOGY CARE	27

    Critical Decision Support, 27

Applying a Human-Centered Design Approach to
 Improving EHR Systems, 32
Integration and Interoperability to Improve EHR
 Functionality and Support a Learning Health
 Care System, 37

IMPROVING EHR DATA COLLECTION TO SUPPORT
CLINICAL CARE, QUALITY AND VALUE, AND RESEARCH   38
Improving Data Collection and Display to Support Clinical
 Decision Making, 38
Opportunities to Improve the Usability of EHRs for Research
 Purposes, 41
Opportunities to Improve EHR Data Collection to Support
 High-Quality Care and Value, 42
Suggestions to Improve Data Collection and Promote
 Data Sharing, 42

FEDERAL AGENCIES AS PARTNERS IN DRIVING
EHR INNOVATION   43
OSTP: The Role of Science and Technology Policy in
 Advancing EHRs, 43
The NCI: Using EHR Data for Cancer Surveillance, 44
The CDC: Leveraging EHRs for Public Health Planning and Research, 46
The FDA: Using EHR Data to Generate Evidence for Oncology
 Product Development, 47
ONC: Advancing Interoperability and Innovation in
 Health IT, 49
CMS: Enabling EHRs to Better Support Health Care Data
 Exchange, 49
Addressing the Challenges of Integrating SDOH Data in
 the EHR, 51
Coordinating EHR-Related Efforts across Federal Agencies
 and with Partners, 52

REFLECTIONS   53
REFERENCES   54

APPENDIX A   STATEMENT OF TASK   59
APPENDIX B   WORKSHOP AGENDA   61

Boxes, Figures, and Table

BOXES

1 Observations on the Current Capabilities and Use of EHRs in Cancer Care: Highlights of Points Made by Individual Workshop Participants, 2
2 Suggestions from Individual Workshop Participants to Advance the Development, Implementation, and Use of EHRs in Oncology Care, Research, and Surveillance, 5

FIGURES

1 Average number of secure patient portal messages per month for the hematology–oncology clinicians at the University of Pennsylvania, 11
2 EHRs in prospective clinical research, 16
3 Integrating patient self-reporting of symptoms into the EHR workflow, 20
4 Spectrum of nudge interventions for clinicians and patients, 24
5 Human-centered approach to EHR design, 32
6 Systems Engineering Initiative for Patient Safety (SEIPS) 3.0 model of patient care, 35
7 Flow of data to the CDC National Program of Cancer Registries, 46

TABLE

1 Framework for a Patient's Health Care Responsibilities and Challenges and Their Impact on Daily Life, 34

Acronyms and Abbreviations

AI	artificial intelligence
AMIA	American Medical Informatics Association
AIMS	APHL's Informatics Messaging Services
APHL	Association of Public Health Laboratories
API	application programming interface
APM	alternative payment models
ASCO	American Society of Clinical Oncology
CDC	Centers for Disease Control and Prevention
CEHRT	certified EHR technology
CMMI	Center for Medicare and Medicaid Innovation
CMS	Centers for Medicare & Medicaid Services
CPT	current procedural terminology
CRISS	Center for Research and Innovation in System Safety
CTAC	Clinical and Translational Research Advisory Committee
EHR	electronic health record
ePRO	electronic patient-reported outcome
FDA	U.S. Food and Drug Administration
FHIR	Fast Healthcare Interoperability Resources
HIE	health information exchange
HIPAA	Health Insurance Portability and Accountability Act of 1996

HITECH	Health Information Technology for Economic and Clinical Health Act
HL7	Health Level 7
ICD	International Classification of Disease
KP	Kaiser Permanente
mCODE	minimal Common Oncology Data Elements
MIPS	Merit-Based Incentive Payment System
ML	machine learning
NCI	National Cancer Institute
NIH	National Institutes of Health
NLP	natural language processing
OHDSI	Observational Health Data Sciences and Informatics
ONC	Office of the National Coordinator for Health Information Technology
OSTP	Office of Science and Technology Policy
PRO	patient-reported outcome
QI	quality improvement
SDOH	social determinants of health
SEER	Surveillance, Epidemiology, and End Results
SEIPS	Systems Engineering Initiative for Patient Safety
SIC	serious illness conversation
USCDI	United States Core Data for Interoperability

Proceedings of a Workshop

WORKSHOP OVERVIEW[1]

On February 28 and March 1, 2022, the National Cancer Policy Forum and the Computer Science and Telecommunications Board of the National Academies of Sciences, Engineering, and Medicine hosted a public workshop to examine opportunities to improve patient care and outcomes through collaborations to enhance innovation in the development, implementation, and use of electronic health records (EHRs) in oncology care, research, and surveillance.

This virtual workshop featured presentations and panel discussions on a range of topics, including

- optimizing the functionality and usability of EHRs in oncology care;
- standardization of oncology EHR documentation to facilitate care and communication between clinicians and patients;
- enhancing EHR structure, data standardization, and interoperability to improve care and enable real-world data collection and sharing for research, surveillance, and quality improvement;

---

[1] This workshop was organized by an independent planning committee whose role was limited to identification of topics and speakers. This Proceedings of a Workshop was prepared by the rapporteurs as a factual summary of the presentations and discussions that took place at the workshop. Statements, recommendations, and opinions expressed are those of individual presenters and participants and are not endorsed or verified by the National Academies of Sciences, Engineering, and Medicine, and they should not be construed as reflecting any group consensus.

- integrating patient-reported outcome (PRO) measures into EHRs; and
- aligning incentives to ensure that EHRs offered by vendors meet the needs of the various users in oncology.

This Proceedings of a Workshop summarizes the presentations and discussions that took place at the workshop. Observations and suggestions from individual participants are discussed throughout the proceedings and highlights are presented in Boxes 1 and 2. (Box 1 includes observations on the current capabilities and use of EHRs in cancer care, and Box 2 outlines potential strategies for advancing the development, implementation, and use of EHRs in oncology care, research, and surveillance.) Appendix A includes the Statement of Task for the workshop. The workshop agenda is provided in Appendix B. Presentations and the workshop webcast have been archived online.[2]

---

[2] See https://www.nationalacademies.org/event/02-28-2022/innovation-in-electronic-health-records-for-oncology-care-research-and-surveillance-a-workshop (accessed May 18, 2022).

BOX 1
Observations on the Current Capabilities and Use of EHRs in Cancer Care:
Highlights of Points Made by Individual Workshop Participants

Clinical Workflow
- EHRs are a significant advance over paper records. They have evolved beyond their original uses for billing and scheduling to serve a broad range of purposes and users, including patients. (Hripcsak, Levy, Shulman)
- EHR-related tasks are not well integrated into clinical workflows, and there is increasing administrative and documentation burden on clinicians, especially for complex diseases such as cancer. (Hripcsak, Russo, Shulman, Zon)
- EHR systems could be better designed to facilitate patient care, but many clinicians voice concern that they interfere with patient care and contribute to clinician burnout. (Hripcsak, Russo, Shulman, Zon)
- Elements are continually added to EHR systems as they evolve (e.g., to incorporate new guidelines, diagnostics, therapies, regulations, or requirements), but elements are

BOX 1 Continued

rarely—if ever—removed, even when they become obsolete. (Hripcsak, Shulman)
- Clinical pathways embedded within EHRs can support care workflows through functionality that displays "the right information at the right time" (e.g., the "hover-to-discover" feature in the Kaiser Permanente Oncology Pathways). (Ichiuji, Malin)
- Both the clinician- and patient-facing interfaces of EHRs are being used to "nudge" evidence-based care. (Meropol, Takvorian, Yabroff)
- Cancer care is provided by teams that are dynamic and fluid (across systems, locations, time) and include individuals who interact with EHRs at different levels. (Carayon, Malin)

EHR Data
- EHRs contain volumes of potentially useful information, but data are often not standardized or are entered as unstructured data, hindering retrievability and exchange of data across systems within an institution and externally. (Haddad, Kluetz, Meropol, Osterman, Penberthy, Shulman, Strawbridge)
- Data in EHRs are of inconsistent quality and are often incomplete, due in part to the fractured nature of the U.S. health care system. (Kluetz, Penberthy, Strawbridge, Warner)
- Efforts to aggregate EHR data often result in data gaps and missing information, partly due to clinician recording of critical data elements in an unstructured, text-based format in the clinical note. (Bertagnolli, Shulman)
- Medical students and oncology residents are trained in problem-oriented clinical documentation for providing care but are generally not trained in EHR documentation more broadly (e.g., translation of clinical notes for lay audiences, use of supportive and inclusive language, entering structured data). (Levy, Patel, Warner)
- Critical data needed for clinical decision making can be difficult to find in the EHR and need to be more prominently and clearly displayed, unobstructed by less critical data, with an understanding that essential data elements can vary by clinical specialty. (Anders, Carayon, Shulman)

continued

BOX 1 Continued

- EHRs are a valuable source of real-world patient data that can support many uses (e.g., care, risk stratification, quality improvement efforts, research, surveillance). (Basch, Kluetz, Meropol, Russo, Shulman)
- Data sharing efforts can be inhibited due to concerns about ownership, patient privacy, and data security. (Tuckson, Warner)
- Collective will and policy change are needed to drive the adoption of standardized data formats and structured data collection to enable the entry of data into the EHR once for use across multiple purposes (e.g., decision support, quality improvement efforts, research). (Levy, Shulman)

Patients and the EHR
- The Federal Interoperability and Information Blocking rule[a] has created opportunities to improve patient-centered care while also creating challenges, including increased documentation burden, as well as concerns about the timing of information release, contributing to patient worry. (Osterman, Patel, Yabroff)
- Patients may face barriers to accessing and understanding the information in their EHR due to a lack of internet access and/or a computer or mobile device, difficulty working with the technology, or low health literacy, which may exacerbate disparities in care and patient outcomes. (Darien, Hughes-Halbert, Osterman, Takvorian)
- Patient-centered communication among clinicians, the patient, and the EHR creates a foundation for trust and patient-centered care. Language used in the EHR that is inflammatory or judgmental can erode trust and can perpetuate biases and stigma, which can adversely affect the delivery of high-quality care. (Darien, Hughes-Halbert, Patel, Shulman)
- The patient experience across the cancer care continuum is different from their care pathway that is documented in the EHR, and EHRs could better capture information about the patient experience. (Malin, Mynatt, Takvorian)
- Integrating patient-reported outcomes (PROs) in the EHR can inform patient management, population health, and quality improvement efforts, as well as provide real-world data for research and policy, but

BOX 1 Continued

there are financial challenges to integrating PROs within EHRs. (Basch, Yabroff)
- The health data in EHRs belong to patients, and any secondary uses of those data need to prioritize providing a benefit to patients. (Bertagnolli, Darien, Shulman, Strawbridge)

---

[a] See https://www.healthit.gov/curesrule/download (accessed August 17, 2022).
NOTE: This list is the rapporteurs' synopsis of observations made by one or more individual speakers as identified. These statements have not been endorsed or verified by the National Academies of Sciences, Engineering, and Medicine. They are not intended to reflect a consensus among workshop participants.

BOX 2
Suggestions from Individual Workshop Participants to Advance the Development, Implementation, and Use of EHRs in Oncology Care, Research, and Surveillance

Developing Critical Features of Next-generation Oncology EHRs
- Prioritize patient-centeredness and create opportunities for greater patient engagement in care decisions. (Basch, Patel, Takvorian, Yabroff)
- Facilitate cancer prevention and cancer screening. (Hripcsak)
- Minimize clinical documentation burden on oncology clinicians. (Basch, Hripcsak, Osterman, Shulman, Takvorian)
- Use data science principles for interpretation of EHR data. (Hripcsak)
- Enable interoperability and data exchange across health systems. (Osterman)
- Inform and support learning health care systems. (Bertagnolli, Levy, Zon)

Improving Functionality of Oncology EHRs
- Conduct and publish pragmatic studies to evaluate current EHR systems to understand the extent to which they facilitate or hinder the clinician experience, the patient

continued

BOX 2 Continued

experience, and patient-clinician communication. (Shulman, Takvorian)
- When designing and implementing new EHR features, assess their potential disadvantages to ensure that adaptations support—not impede—high-quality care (e.g., additional "clicks" needed to complete a task in the EHR). (Hripcsak, Ichiuji, Russo, Shulman, Takvorian, Yabroff)
- Employ a sociotechnical systems approach to EHR design to create a collaborative EHR environment for information exchange and to account for differences in how individuals interact with technology. (Carayon, Malin)
- Integrate formalized cancer pathways into the EHR, but allow for deviation/customization by the clinician. (Malin, Zon)
- Document deviations from cancer pathways to support a learning health care system and enable refinement of pathways. (Anders, Malin, Zon)
- Provide incentives from payers for integration of oncology clinical pathways across practices and EHR systems. (Malin, Zon)
- Pursue innovation in clinical decision support, such as embedding computable cancer screening guidelines. (Dowling, Richardson)
- Identify and collect the information most needed by the end users of EHR data, including clinicians and patients (e.g., critical data for shared decision making, information on social determinants of health). (Anders, Dowling, Haddad, Hughes-Halbert, Kluetz, Sim)
- Improve the capture, retrievability, and sharing of health data across health care systems:
  - Develop capabilities to extract structured data from unstructured EHR information, including natural language processing (NLP),[a] artificial intelligence (AI),[b] and machine-learning (ML)[c] algorithms. (Dowling, Haddad, Hughes-Halbert, Meropol, Penberthy, Warner)
  - Systematically capture PROs. (Basch, Haddad, Warner)
  - Pursue improvements in EHR interoperability and data standardization. (Bertagnolli, Dowling, Haddad, Ichiuji, Mynatt, Shanbhag, Strawbridge, Zon)
- Facilitate use of EHR data for cancer surveillance. (Dowling, Penberthy)

Enhancing Collaboration
- Collaborate with technology vendors to ensure that NLP and ML algorithms and models are inclusive of diverse populations. (Haddad, Strawbridge)
- Collaborate with human-centered design experts and systems engineers to revamp the clinical workflow and develop health IT technology that fits that workflow, rather than forcing workflows to bend to the technology. (Anders, Haddad, Strawbridge)
- Partner with payers around the shared goal of high-quality, efficient care. (Strawbridge, Tuckson)
- Engage intergovernmental and other collaborators to define the data that different end users need from the EHR. (Anders, Kluetz, Sim)

Improving Policy
- Revisit the regulations promulgated under HIPAA that impact the sharing and use of data in the EHR. (Strawbridge, Tuckson, Warner)
- Build a national health data sharing platform to leverage the full potential of EHR-based, real-world data for patient care and research. Develop a standard data set and interface and incentivize participation. (Meropol, Russo, Strawbridge)
- Coordinate efforts across federal agencies and with state, tribal, local, and territorial partners, industry, and academia. (Dowling, Sim)

---

[a] Natural language processing (NLP) "is a branch of artificial intelligence that helps computers understand, interpret and manipulate human language. NLP draws from many disciplines, including computer science and computational linguistics, in its pursuit to fill the gap between human communication and computer understanding." See https://www.sas.com/en_us/insights/analytics/what-is-natural-language-processing-nlp.html (accessed October 13, 2022).

[b] Artificial intelligence (AI) refers to "systems or machines that mimic human intelligence to perform tasks and can iteratively improve themselves based on the information they collect." See https://www.oracle.com/artificial-intelligence/what-is-ai/ (accessed October 13, 2022).

[c] Machine learning (ML) is "a subfield of artificial intelligence that gives computers the ability to learn without explicitly being programmed." See https://mitsloan.mit.edu/ideas-made-to-matter/machine-learning-explained (accessed October 13, 2022).

NOTE: This list is the rapporteurs' synopsis of suggestions made by one or more individual speakers as identified. These statements have not been endorsed or verified by the National Academies of Sciences, Engineering, and Medicine. They are not intended to reflect a consensus among workshop participants.

OVERVIEW OF THE USE OF EHRS IN ONCOLOGY CARE, RESEARCH, AND SURVEILLANCE

"When we talk about electronic health records . . . we're actually talking about hundreds of systems that are integrated together," said Mia Levy, chief medical officer at Foundation Medicine. She provided an overview of current and emerging elements of EHRs:

- **Transaction systems** Early EHRs were often transaction systems supporting billing and scheduling, Levy said.
- **Clinical documentation systems** EHRs evolved to include clinical documentation that mirrored the traditional patient chart, supporting ordering, displaying results and reports, and facilitating the creation of clinical notes.
- **Patient safety systems** Following publication of the Institute of Medicine consensus study, *To Err is Human: Building a Safer Health System* (2000), EHRs began to focus on quality and safety. Patient-safety systems were designed to help reduce medical errors through tools such as decision-support systems, barcoded medication administration, and specimen barcoding, Levy said.
- **Specialty-specific and disease-specific subsystems** Examples of specialty-specific EHR subsystems important for oncology care include radiology, laboratory, and radiation oncology systems. Cancer-specific subsystems include, for example, chemotherapy treatment management systems, cancer staging systems, and oncology history modules. Levy said that vendors and health care organizations can face challenges balancing the competing needs and priorities of the enterprise EHR system and disease- or specialty-specific subsystems with regard to the development of features within the applications.
- **Longitudinal treatment plan management** Another important EHR feature for oncology care is longitudinal management of the patient treatment plan. This includes, for example, automated medication dose calculations, complex treatment scheduling and medication sequencing, and integrated safety checks, as well as access to libraries of standard-of-care treatment protocols and clinical trial protocols. Levy said it would be helpful to collaborate across institutions to develop decision support for longitudinal treatment plan management because protocol libraries are usually maintained by staff at each institution, resulting in substantial duplication of effort.
- **Communication systems** EHRs now incorporate asynchronous messaging platforms that facilitate communication, both among health care team members and between the patient and their care teams,

that complies with the Privacy Rule promulgated under the Health Insurance Portability and Accountability Act of 1996 (HIPAA).[3] Levy described the current level of communication through these systems as "astronomical." For example, a study estimated there were 1.9 messages for the oncologist and 3.5 for the oncology nurse associated with each ambulatory patient appointment (Steitz and Levy, 2017). Levy added that instant messaging is replacing phone calls and pages for real-time communications among the care team, and there has been significant uptake of asynchronous communication between patients and their care team during the COVID-19 pandemic.

- **Patient engagement** Patients can now access a personal health record, tethered to their EHR at a particular institution, where they can monitor their health using devices (e.g., glucose levels, blood pressure), and they can share their health information with their care team or researchers as electronic patient-reported outcomes (ePROs).
- **Health information exchange (HIE)** Levy said that HIE occurs when EHR systems facilitate the direct sharing of patient health records, which is "a vital part of decreasing health care costs and improving the quality of care." She noted that there is still much work to be done to enable interoperability across health systems.
- **Telehealth** The uptake of telehealth for patient care that does not require an inpatient visit expanded dramatically during the COVID-19 pandemic, Levy said.
- **Research systems** Clinical information systems are starting to be leveraged to support research activities, such as clinical trial matching, participant enrollment, completion of case report forms, toxicity reporting, clinical outcomes reporting, and clinical trial billing compliance.
- **Mobile systems** Clinicians can now access a patient's EHR remotely through mobile systems.
- **Continuous learning health care system** Together, these many systems can help to achieve the vision of a continuous learning health care system, Levy said.

The EHR in Clinical Oncology Practice

Oncology is a high-risk, high-stakes, time-pressured practice that is increasing in clinical complexity and administrative burden, said Lawrence Shulman, professor of medicine and deputy director for clinical services at the University

---

[3] See https://www.hhs.gov/hipaa/for-professionals/privacy/index.html (accessed August 17, 2022).

of Pennsylvania Abramson Cancer Center. Oncologists strive to provide safe, high-quality cancer care in the face of these clinical and systemic complexities.

Recalling the days of paper charts, Shulman said that today's oncologists "spend [their] clinical lives in the EHR." He described some of the limitations of current EHRs that negatively affect a clinician's daily work: EHRs are generally designed to serve all specialties, so there is limited specialization of the EHR; they are primarily designed for billing and compliance purposes; volumes of data from many different contributors can be very "messy" and difficult to interpret; and critical data needed for decision making are often difficult to find or missing. Shulman observed that EHRs have become increasingly burdensome for clinicians as elements are continually added to meet complex regulatory and institutional requirements and to incorporate new diagnostics, therapies, and guidelines. However, he said, few data elements are ever removed, such that clinicians face a daunting workload of EHR-related tasks. "Systems must support, not thwart, high-quality care," he said.

Drawing on the work of Atul Gawande (2004), Shulman said that "medical outcomes are the sum of many parts," and that quality stems from the convergence of people and systems, including EHRs. In 2018, Gawande described his personal experience with EHRs, saying "I've come to feel that a system that promised to increase my mastery over my work has, instead, increased my work's mastery over me," and he wrote about a colleague who described her EHR in-basket as "clogged to the point of dysfunction." Shulman said the hematology–oncology practices at his institution currently receive, on average, more than 160 secure patient portal messages per hematologist/oncologist each month through the EHR system (Figure 1). One recent study found that physicians spend 5.5 hours in the EHR for every eight hours of clinic time (Melnick et al., 2021), and Shulman added that many of his physician colleagues complete their clinic notes at home, after their children are asleep.

Shulman discussed how, in the cockpit design of modern passenger jets, all instruments are readily accessible but only the instruments showing the most critical data are directly in front of the pilots. He suggested that a similar approach is needed for how EHRs display data if they are to support safe and effective oncology care. He argued that critical patient data be "unencumbered by unneeded information, . . . maximally accessible, [and] . . . displayed without ambiguity," adding that longitudinal displays be available when relevant. Critical data for oncology clinicians include, for example, cancer staging; the longitudinal cancer course; and pathology, radiology, and laboratory findings. Shulman suggested that a "shell" could be created over the EHR, which would summarize the impressions from different imaging procedures or pathology reports, for example, so that the key information would be more readily accessible, with a link to the full report.

"The oncology careforce is under tremendous pressure," Shulman said. He

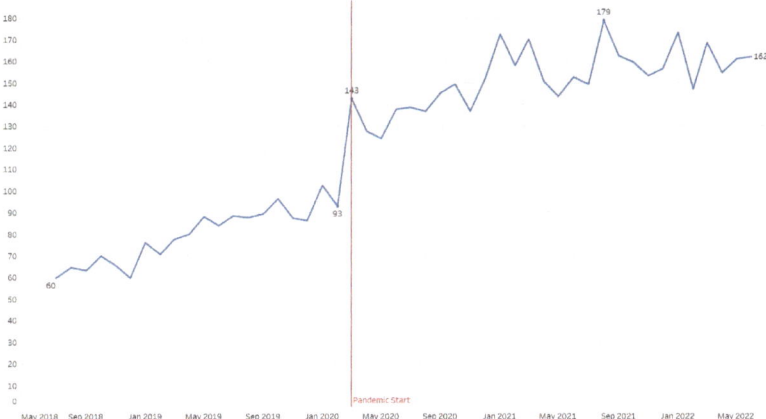

FIGURE 1 Average number of secure patient portal messages per month for the hematology–oncology clinicians at the University of Pennsylvania. The number of messages increased substantially after the onset of the COVID-19 pandemic.
SOURCE: Shulman presentation, February 28, 2022. Graphic designed by Peter Gabriel.

suggested that increasing the efficiency of oncology care by improving the functionality and efficiency of EHRs "may be the only solution that will allow clinicians to care for more patients without extending work hours" (Shulman et al., 2020; see also NASEM 2019). He described how experts in process improvement shadowed the oncologists at the University of Pennsylvania to understand how they interacted physically with the EHR as they provided care to patients in the clinic. They found that care and EHR tasks were "disjointed," and he said there is much room for improvement. Shulman and other workshop participants urged EHR vendors to be engaged in efforts to improve EHRs to foster improved usability and integration within care workflows. Levy noted that the workflow is "people, process, and technology. The EHR in isolation isn't the problem alone."

The EHR and the Patient's Relationship with Health Care Providers

The EHR is a powerful tool that can either facilitate or impede trust, patient–clinician communication, and improved patient outcomes, depending on how it is used, said Gwen Darien, executive vice president for patient advocacy engagement at the National Patient Advocate Foundation. As a three-time cancer survivor, she emphasized the need for bidirectional trust between patients and their care providers and the importance of seeing the patient as a person, not simply as data embedded in an EHR on the computer screen.

Bidirectional Patient–Clinician Communication

From a communication perspective, Darien said that it is important for EHRs and patient portals to be transparent and foster trust. Patients reading their EHR often find that the clinical notes do not reflect their conversations with their clinician, which she said undermines trust in the clinician and the care they provide. For example, Darien described being very disturbed that the clinical notes in her EHR about the possibility of her cancer recurring were different from what her clinician communicated at the visit.

The language used when recording clinical observations can also perpetuate biases, influencing how patients are perceived by subsequent clinicians and how patients see themselves and their conditions. This includes racially and ethnically biased language, as well as potentially judgmental or inflammatory language, such as describing a patient as noncompliant or nonadherent without any notation as to why the patient did not complete a particular aspect of the care plan. Darien urged clinicians to write clinical documentation in the EHR with the expectation that patients and their families will read it. Chanita Hughes-Halbert, associate director for cancer equity at the University of Southern California Norris Comprehensive Cancer Center and professor and vice chair for research in the Department of Population and Public Health Sciences, added that the use of biased language can affect the quality of care a patient receives, citing a study showing that stigmatizing language was more frequently used in EHRs of Black patients compared to White patients (Himmelstein et al., 2022).

Darien said that the medical record is a tool to enable the patient to work with their care team to co-plan their health care strategy. She said that one strategy to promote patient-centered communication and build bidirectional trust is for clinicians and patients to look at the patient information on the computer screen together during the appointment, creating what physician Maria Alkureishi has described as a "triangle of trust" (Alkureishi et al., 2021).

Many workshop speakers discussed reimagining clinical documentation, given that patients are now a primary user of the EHR. Levy said physicians are trained in problem-oriented documentation, which uses complex clinical terminology because it was originally intended for use only by health care professionals managing patient care. Today, through the Open Notes[4] movement, patients have access to all their medical records. In response, many institutions have added disclaimers warning that the clinical notes are "written by doctors for doctors" in language that patients might not be able to easily understand, and clinicians are increasingly spending visit time interpreting these notes for patients.

Hughes-Halbert said there is inherent tension with the language used in EHRs: Problem-oriented documentation might still be necessary for clinical

---

[4] See https://www.opennotes.org/ (accessed August 17, 2022).

team member communication, while patient users of the EHR may require more understandable—and less anxiety-provoking—language. She suggested that patients and clinicians work collaboratively to develop a system that better serves the needs of all users. Shulman agreed and said that, ideally, health care is a "joint effort" between clinicians and their patient, and the EHR is one component of that team-based work. He noted that different health care professionals have different levels of interaction with the EHR and the patient. For example, a radiologist who reviews and interprets a CT scan or X-ray might never meet the patient or know the context of their overall care plan, unlike their oncologist. Neal Meropol, vice president of research oncology at Flatiron Health, recalled that when patient portals were first launched, there were some concerns about patients seeing their clinical results before the physician could discuss the clinical significance of the results. However, he said there was general agreement that promoting patient access to medical records would improve patient–clinician communication. The challenge is how to efficiently communicate clinical information—in part by leveraging the EHR—so that this information does not cause undue anxiety or create confusion.

Levy noted that an after-visit summary is intended to be written in patient-centered language, but clinicians are not trained in translating clinical notes for lay use. The question is how to minimize the burden of this added documentation for clinicians while still providing useful information to patients.

Patient Access to Their EHR

"Unequal access and treatment persist despite—or because of—the medium of health care encounters," Darien said. For example, the COVID-19 pandemic facilitated the expansion of telehealth for patients. But Darien pointed out that many patients face barriers to receiving telehealth services, such as lack of a private place to conduct the appointment or lack of reliable phone or internet connectivity. Similarly, a patient may be unable to view their patient portal due to a lack of a computer, smartphone, or broadband internet service. Hughes-Halbert said that a recent survey found that disparities in access to a traditional computer and to home broadband internet persist,[5] highlighting these disparities as a social justice issue.

---

[5] See https://www.pewresearch.org/internet/fact-sheet/internet-broadband/?menuItem=3109350c-8dba-4b7f-ad52-a3e976ab8c8f (accessed May 18, 2022).

Integrating Social Determinants of Health in EHRs

Hughes-Halbert said that a person's health is influenced by the social determinants of health (SDOH), or the conditions in which they live, learn, work, and play (e.g., housing, neighborhood, food security, education, access to high-quality health care).[6] She noted that health care systems are increasingly taking SDOH into account in health care delivery and research and are looking at ways to document SDOH in EHRs.

Hughes-Halbert said the Medical University of South Carolina Transdisciplinary Collaborative Center in Precision Medicine and Minority Men's Health is developing tools and resources to integrate data on SDOH with clinical information, including the development of natural language processing (NLP) tools that can extract narrative information on SDOH from the EHR. She noted that the Center is also considering the ethical, legal, and social implications associated with EHR documentation of SDOH. For example, using a NLP tool, researchers were able extract from the clinical notes in EHRs information on social isolation and loneliness in patients with prostate cancer (Zhu et al., 2019), but Hughes-Halbert noted that some of the language that clinicians used to document social isolation could be considered stigmatizing or could be potentially offensive to a patient reading their chart. In another study of patients with prostate cancer, Hughes-Halbert and colleagues demonstrated the association of social deprivation with disparities in patient portal activation and research participation (Hughes-Halbert et al., 2021).

Meropol and Hughes-Halbert discussed the potential of data linkages to compensate for a lack of clinician documentation of SDOH in the EHR. For example, Meropol said, census block–level data on SDOH could be used as a proxy for individual patient information on SDOH. Hughes-Halbert agreed, but cautioned that area-level or community-level measures, while useful, do not necessarily reflect a given individual's lived experience within that area. Additionally, some SDOH information that could be incorporated within the EHR may exceed the level of personal information a patient wants to share with their clinician. Darien said that some patients fear that disclosing certain information about themselves will affect the quality of care they receive. In her prior conversations with patients and patient advocates about the cost of care, patients expressed concern about being profiled and said they did not want to share information about their finances or, in some cases, even their address with their clinicians. Shulman said this highlights the importance of personalization of health care infrastructure, including EHRs, based on patient preferences.

---

[6] See https://www.thenationshealth.org/content/infographics-social-determinants-health (accessed May 18, 2022).

"Continued efforts are needed to understand the effects of multilevel social determinants on cancer health disparities," Hughes-Halbert said. She suggested collecting information on SDOH in EHRs and evaluating interventions to address SDOH to assess their impact on cancer care and patient outcomes.

The EHR in Quality Improvement and Research

Quality improvement (QI) in health care entails a cycle of defining a set of quality metrics, introducing performance-improvement interventions, and measuring performance against the metrics, said Meropol. The findings are then used to refine the metrics and/or interventions, while continuing to measure performance. Quality improvement programs are also informed by the outputs of research (e.g., evidence-based interventions and best practices, quality metrics and performance measures, benchmarking).

Although EHRs were not originally intended to support QI or research, Meropol said they are adaptable for these purposes because EHRs are a rich resource of patient-level information from multiple data sources. All patients in a clinical practice have an EHR, and data are generally collected in real time as part of the point-of-care workflow and stored in a digital format. When using the data in EHRs for QI and research, Meropol said the necessary components include a framework for patient privacy, curation capabilities for structured and unstructured data, front-end and back-end access[7] to the EHR, and linkages to data outside the EHR. He also emphasized that machine learning (ML) and NLP tools can be applied, with the goal of ensuring that data are interpretable, reliable, and unbiased.

Cancer care QI initiatives that are or could be enabled by EHRs include measurement of concordance with clinical practice guidelines and quality metrics, benchmarking, treatment decision support, risk prediction modeling, and prompts or nudges for clinicians (e.g., to order a diagnostic test or document particular information). Meropol added that EHR data are also being used by platforms such as Patients Like Mine (Gombar et al., 2019), which enable clinicians to see real-time information about other similar patients to inform clinical decision making.

Meropol said that EHRs have applicability for retrospective research because they are a robust source of real-world data, noting that EHR data have been used to study practice patterns and patient outcomes, health care disparities, and comparative effectiveness analyses; to support regulatory decision making; and to inform the design of prospective studies. Some limitations of using

---

[7] Front-end use of EHRs includes groups such as clinicians and patients, while the back-end use includes groups such as researchers, developers, and other experts in health informatics who need access to the databases where EHR data are stored.

EHR data for retrospective research include missing data, the potential for bias, inadequate collection of patient outcomes data, inconsistent documentation of patient exposures, and challenges in assessing causal inference, he said. One way to reduce missing data is to intentionally collect data for key parameters needed to address research questions, such as adverse events or imaging at specific time points. In other words, Meropol said, prospective evidence generation can be built upon the platform of routinely collected real-world data.

Meropol discussed a range of opportunities for leveraging EHRs across the lifecycle of prospective clinical research to increase efficiency and reduce the operational burden on clinical trial sites (Figure 2). For example, EHR data collected during routine care can inform trial design, support point-of-care patient ascertainment and randomization, and assist with study site selection. Meropol advocated for "implement[ing] pragmatic study design elements and leveraging routinely collected data whenever possible." He added that integrating clinical research into routine clinical care can help to facilitate inclusion of more diverse, representative populations in cancer research.

Meropol said that most of the data in EHRs is unstructured. Algorithms are helpful for extracting and interpreting unstructured data but, he said, human involvement is always required, whether for developing the algorithms or interpreting the outputs. He suggested that more structured data be collected within EHRs in order to improve the functionality of EHR data for downstream users (e.g., clinical care, research, QI). He called for improved interoperability of EHR systems and added that the adoption of common data standards would help facilitate the collection of data from different EHR systems for activities such as research, QI, or benchmarking.

Meropol noted that the Food and Drug Administration (FDA) has provided guidance on opportunities to use real-world evidence, including EHR data,

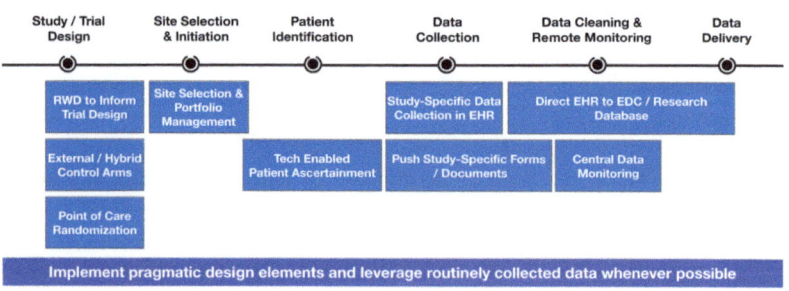

FIGURE 2 EHRs in prospective clinical research.
NOTES: RWD = real-world data; EDC = electronic data capture.
SOURCE: Meropol presentation, February 28, 2022.

in regulatory decision-making.[8] Recent recommendations from the National Cancer Institute (NCI) Clinical and Translational Research Advisory Committee (CTAC) focused on the use of EHRs to improve the conduct of clinical trials.[9] To achieve the goal of having an integrated EHR-based evidence generation platform and QI system, Meropol stressed that the clinical and research communities will need to "incentivize high-quality data entry, legislate interoperability, promote adoption of data standards, and normalize data sharing with appropriate privacy protections."

IMPROVING THE PATIENT-FACING ASPECTS OF EHRs

As previously discussed, patients are a key user of the EHR. Many workshop speakers discussed opportunities to improve patient-facing aspects of the EHR to enable patient–clinician communication with the goal of improving cancer care and patient outcomes.

Today's Patient Portal

"Today's patient portal looks very different than the patient portal of even just two or three years ago," said Travis Osterman, assistant professor of biomedical informatics and hematology and oncology, and the director of Cancer Clinical Informatics at the Vanderbilt-Ingram Cancer Center. In recent decades, health care systems have provided patients with some degree of access to their personal health record via patient portals that are accessible through a website or mobile application. Osterman said this was generally "a very small piece of the medical record, or a redacted view." This changed in 2021, with the implementation of the Interoperability and Information Blocking rule promulgated under the 21st Century Cures Act.[10]

Jyoti Patel, medical director of thoracic oncology and assistant director for clinical research at the Robert H. Lurie Comprehensive Cancer Center of Northwestern University, explained that under this rule, it is now legally required that patients be provided with immediate access to all the health information in their EHR. This includes information such as consultation notes, discharge summaries, progress notes, imaging narratives, laboratory and pathology reports, and procedure notes. Certain mental health records are excluded, and certain information may also be withheld due to privacy or security concerns, or to

---

[8] See https://www.fda.gov/science-research/science-and-research-special-topics/real-world-evidence (accessed May 18, 2022).

[9] See https://deainfo.nci.nih.gov/advisory/ctac/1120/SPWGreport.pdf (accessed May 18, 2022).

[10] See https://www.healthit.gov/curesrule/download (accessed August 17, 2022).

prevent potential harm. Osterman added that the rule also includes provisions to address information blocking, or impeding patient access to this information.

The EHR as a Tool for Patient–Clinician Communication

Providing understandable information in the EHR is an "opportunity to extend the visit," Patel said, and evidence suggests that providing patients access to their EHR improves communication, treatment adherence, and patient outcomes. Data also suggest that using supportive language and avoiding stigmatizing language helps to promote trust between patients and clinicians. In a survey of patients undergoing radiation therapy, most (greater than 90 percent) felt that having access to their clinical notes gave them a better understanding of their diagnosis and the risks and side effects of their treatments and provided information they had missed during the in-person visit. However, some patients reported they felt more worried (11 percent) or more confused (6 percent) after reading their notes, and 4 percent of those surveyed said they regretted having read the notes (Shaverdian et al., 2019).

Clinicians have also expressed some concerns about these changes. In a survey of oncologists and non-oncology physicians, approximately 70 percent in both groups responded that the sharing of clinical notes with patients would lead them to be to less candid in documenting their patient's diagnosis and prognosis (McCleary et al., 2018). Similarly, in another survey, oncologists who shared clinical notes with their patients reported spending more time writing notes and being more restrictive in the information they included. The oncologists were "moderately positive" about the impact of open access to EHRs, Patel said, responding that sharing clinical notes was helpful and that patients were more prepared for their clinic visits, but that most patients were more worried than before (Moll and Cajander, 2020).

With the instantaneous electronic delivery of results, patients are regularly seeing results before the clinician, often in medical jargon patients may not understand and without context, Patel said, resulting in clinicians spending a lot of appointment time "justifying the language and explaining the clinical significance." Patel shared several examples from her own practice of patients with cancer who experienced distress when viewing results that were posted in their patient portal prior to their appointment. She said patients who were undergoing surveillance imaging learned about a cancer recurrence or new cancers through their EHR, in some cases, on a weekend. Patel described how one patient experienced significant depression and resigned herself to hospice, initially rejecting any discussion of alternative treatment options. Patel said it took concerted effort and time to discuss alternative treatment options. A year later, the patient is doing well on treatment, but is still "angry about the results coming through [the patient portal] and not having a clear path [of care from] the moment that she saw the results," Patel said. She added that common, descriptive imaging terminology in the clinical note can undermine trust because it is unfamiliar and sounds worrisome (e.g., tortuous thoracic aorta, crazy paving pattern in the lung). A family interpreted these distressing terms to mean the cancer was recurring (it was not) and thought Patel had been hiding this from them.

Patel said there are opportunities to improve communication and reduce misunderstandings. She wrote a blog post[11] on Cancer.Net[12] with tips for patients on how to use their portals most effectively and efficiently. Another approach would be to incorporate infographics in the EHR, perhaps "hover boxes [that] could enhance understanding without burdening physicians or compromising the quality of records," said Patel. She also called for oncology clinician education and training to include guidance on using more supportive, inclusive language in their clinical notes.

Osterman drew from a recent editorial by Tempero (2021) to highlight opportunities for clinicians to better communicate with their patients through the EHR:

- **Reduce abbreviations.** Reduce ambiguity by, for example, spelling out "shortness of breath" instead of the abbreviation "SOB," which, Osterman said, might be easily misinterpreted by a nonmedical reader.
- **Stick to the facts.** Avoid speculation or opinion, Osterman said.
- **Remember that the patient will read the record.** Although patients have always had the right to request and receive their medical records, Open Notes now enables them immediate access their full EHR.
- **Set expectations for when results will be posted.** The immediate availability of results such as biopsy or radiology reports showing progression of disease can cause significant patient anxiety, Osterman noted. He suggested that when clinicians order diagnostic testing or imaging during the patient visit, they also set expectations for when they will be available to the patient to discuss the results after they appear in the EHR.

---

[11] See https://www.cancer.net/blog/2021-11/how-make-most-your-patient-portal-during-cancer (accessed May 18, 2022).

[12] In 2002, the American Society of Clinical Oncology (ASCO) launched Cancer.Net to help patients and their caregivers better understand their cancer and better advocate for themselves. See https://www.cancer.net (accessed May 18, 2022).

Integrating Patient-Reported Outcomes into Oncology EHR Systems

Poorly managed symptoms in patients receiving cancer treatment can cause unnecessary discomfort and complications and can lead to emergency room visits and hospitalizations, said Ethan Basch, chief of the Division of Oncology and director of the Lineberger Cancer Outcomes Research Program at the University of North Carolina at Chapel Hill. Although symptom monitoring is an essential component of oncology care, studies have found that clinicians are missing many of the symptoms experienced by their patients undergoing treatment (Basch, 2010).

Integrating patient self-reporting into the EHR workflow could help to identify symptoms early, at a stage where interventions could prevent downstream complications, Basch said. He described how patients could be enrolled in an ePRO program that would send them regular prompts (e.g., weekly) to self-report any symptoms. Real-time alerts are then sent to the patient's care team for further attention and action as needed (Figure 3).

Basch showed several examples of ePRO patient interfaces including a freestanding ePRO system that operates in parallel to (but distinct from) the EHR; a commercial ePRO system that interfaces with a commercial EHR system; and ePRO functionality built within the EHR system. Each system offers various ways for clinicians to visualize data. An advantage of having an ePRO instrument embedded within the EHR is the ability to automatically import PRO data into the clinical notes. Basch showed an example of how the clinician can then use drop-down menus to provide interpretation and note any actions taken in response.

The PRO data in the EHR can be used by clinicians for individual patient management, by patient care coordinators for risk stratification to identify

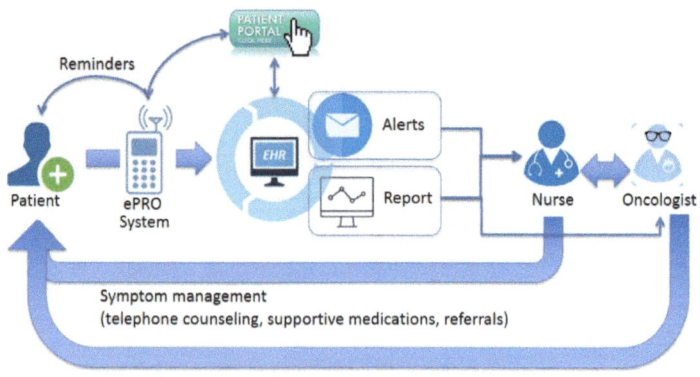

FIGURE 3 Integrating patient self-reporting of symptoms into the EHR workflow.
SOURCE: Basch presentation, February 28, 2022.

patients who would benefit from outreach, by administrators for population health management, by hospitals for quality assessment, and by researchers and payers as a source of real-world data, Basch said. He added that the value of using PROs to help monitor symptoms in clinical oncology practice has been demonstrated by multiple randomized controlled trials and population studies (such as Basch et al., 2017; Denis et al., 2019). Research also supports the feasibility of collecting PROs in clinical practice, with 60 to 80 percent of patients self-reporting when prompted, he said (Basch et al., 2022; Patt et al., 2021).

The ePROs have three key technical functions within the EHR, Basch said—administrative, clinician-facing, and patient-facing tasks. An administrative interface includes a registration system to enroll patients in the ePRO program and a dashboard showing compliance with self-reporting. A clinician interface will provide alert notifications, an audit trail for how alerts are cleared, and the capability to visualize PRO data. A patient interface will send automated prompts to remind patients to self-report, follow up with those who do not respond, and provide access to PRO surveys; it will also send alerts to the clinician when a patient reports severe or worsening symptoms.

The main barriers to integrating ePROs into cancer clinical care are reimbursement and payment challenges, Basch said. He said that the use of new current procedural terminology (CPT) codes for remote therapeutic monitoring is currently restricted to respiratory and musculoskeletal conditions. In addition, reimbursement for ePRO systems requires more frequent transmissions of PRO data per month than is typically needed for use in oncology care. Reimbursement is usually dependent on direct physician supervision, which he said is not practical for how PROs are collected and used in oncology care.

Several workshop speakers discussed opportunities for improving ePRO implementation in cancer care. Basch called for CPT codes to be modified to accommodate the use of ePROs in oncology care. He also noted that the new voluntary cancer payment model from the Centers for Medicare & Medicaid Services (CMS), the Enhancing Oncology Model, will require participating sites to incorporate ePROs for symptom monitoring. Basch also said that the development of standard practices for implementing ePRO systems could help improve usability for clinicians, staff, and patients.

Samuel Takvorian, a genitourinary medical oncologist and assistant professor of medicine at the University of Pennsylvania Perelman School of Medicine, said it is important to "meet patients where they are," especially given their comfort level with the technology used by ePRO systems. He added that clinicians need to communicate to patients that PROs play an important role in their care, and that clinicians will tailor patient care based on the information patients share with the ePRO system. Takvorian also said that while optimal implementation of ePROs can improve clinical workflows, it is important to be aware of unintended consequences that could further increase the burden on clinicians.

Data from wearable devices can also be integrated into the EHR. George Hripcsak, Vivian Beaumont Allen Professor and chair of biomedical informatics at Columbia University and director of Medical Informatics Services for New York Presbyterian Hospital, said that some patients type in their glucose levels manually into their ePRO system because they find it easier than connecting the glucose monitoring device to the PRO application.

Osterman highlighted the need for metadata to accompany the health data being reported from patient devices (e.g., identification of the specific smart devices that collected the data). Without this metadata it becomes difficult to understand how values obtained by different devices and across different health systems truly compare.

Sharing of Patient Data within and among EHR Systems

Regulations promulgated under the 21st Century Cures Act also address the interoperability of EHR systems across health care systems. Osterman said that the Fast Healthcare Interoperability Resources (FHIR) standard facilitates interoperability and exchange of data between health care systems. However, FHIR standards do not cover all data elements in the EHR needed for cancer care delivery. For example, accessible data elements include procedures, medications, lab results, and the care plan; data that are, as yet, inaccessible include chemotherapy dose and cycle, adverse events, metastatic status, and tumor size.

To better enable the capture and sharing of oncology data across systems, Osterman said that a FHIR-based core set of minimal Common Oncology Data Elements (mCODE) is being developed within the data standards structure of HL7 (Health Level Seven, a standard for exchanging information between medical information systems).[13] Oncology data element domains include patient, disease, treatment, outcomes, genomics, and assessment. mCODE will support a standard health record for patients with cancer that will enable information exchange among key participants in cancer care and cancer research, including patients, clinicians, payers, researchers, EHR vendors, and regulators, Osterman said. He added that there is broad community engagement to support the development and implementation of mCODE.[14]

Osterman reviewed some of the key challenges that will need to be addressed to improve data sharing across EHR systems. Greater portability of complex data between systems is needed, he said. For example, patients often bring paper cop-

---

[13] For more information see http://hl7.org/fhir/us/mcode/ (accessed May 18, 2022).

[14] See https://confluence.hl7.org/display/COD/mCODE+Community+of+Practice (accessed May 18, 2022).

ies of their gene sequencing results from outside laboratories to their clinic visit. These reports are scanned into the EHR but in a format that does not readily support clinician decision support. Computable clinical practice guidelines, or having clinical guidelines in a structured format, could help support clinicians by enabling identification of potential treatment options or flagging treatments that deviate from the standard of care, for example. The EHR could also be leveraged to suggest relevant clinical trials for patients, through computable structures for clinical trial inclusion and exclusion criteria.

Using the EHR to Nudge Evidence-Based Cancer Care

"Whether intentional or not, the design of the EHR and its patient-facing applications already affect clinician and patient behavior," Takvorian said. He said there is an opportunity to leverage the EHR as a tool to nudge—or change the way choices are presented that alters behavior predictably but without restricting choice—to improve patient outcomes.[15] In health and health care, for example, a nudge can raise a patient's or clinician's awareness of a choice before them and of the health-related benefits of each choice (e.g., taking the stairs versus the escalator, prescribing a generic versus brand therapy). The design of a nudge can span the spectrum from informational (providing education or feedback) to influential (making the optimal choice the easiest choice) (Figure 4). Takvorian noted that Penn Medicine has a Nudge Unit devoted to designing, implementing, and evaluating nudges to promote evidence-based health care.

Takvorian said nudges in the EHR can promote high-value prescribing practices in both primary care and oncology care settings. For example, generic prescribing rates were increased to more than 95 percent across most drug classes by making the generic equivalent the EHR default choice across the health system, with an opt-out checkbox for "dispense as written" (Patel et al., 2016). EHR-based nudges were also applied to effectively promote the use of more cost-effective options for antiresorptive bone therapies among choices with similar efficacy profiles. Takvorian said the most effective nudge is when there is accountable justification in which prescribers have to defend the need for the less cost-effective option (Takvorian et al., 2020).

EHR-based nudges intended for patients can complement nudges to clinicians, Takvorian said. He described an ongoing study of the impact of patient and clinician nudges on increasing the completion of serious illness conversations (SIC).[16] Clinicians are nudged to conduct a SIC with patients at high risk of mortality who do not have a documented SIC; these same patients are nudged

---

[15] For additional background see Thaler and Sunstein (2009).

[16] "Serious illness conversations (SICs) are an evidence-based approach to eliciting patients' values, goals, and care preferences. Early SICs improve patient outcomes and are recommended

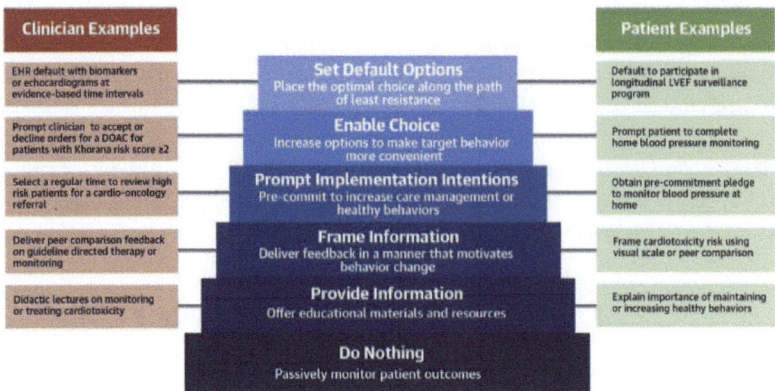

FIGURE 4 Spectrum of nudge interventions for clinicians and patients.
SOURCE: Waddell presentation, February 28, 2022, reprinted from Waddell et al. (2020).

to complete a questionnaire that prepares them to have a SIC with their clinician at a future appointment (Takvorian et al., 2021). He noted the need to rigorously evaluate the findings of pragmatic studies of EHR design elements—including nudges—to understand the impact, identify unintended consequences, and refine as needed.

Next-Generation EHRs

Hripcsak said that today's EHR serves multiple purposes (e.g., clinical care, research, billing) and noted the burden of documentation on clinicians has long been recognized, especially for complex diseases such as cancer (Cusack et al., 2013). He said there are ongoing efforts to address this, including the 25x5 Initiative of the American Medical Informatics Association (AMIA), which aims to reduce the documentation burden by 75 percent in five years;[17] the Observational Health Data Sciences and Informatics (OHDSI) Oncology Working Group project to improve EHR documentation to capture the complexity of cancer progression; and the use of data science to improve information review for patients and clinicians (Hirsch et al., 2015).

Hripcsak said the EHR can be leveraged to engage patients in their care (Prey et al., 2018). Patients are capable of learning to use health monitoring technology for self-management and, as an example, he cited a study in which

---

by national guidelines," Takvorian explained. However, many patients receive end-of-life care that goes against their desires due to lack of a documented SIC.

[17] See https://amia.org/about-amia/amia-25x5 (accessed May 18, 2022).

patients who were unfamiliar with technology learned to reliably self-administer home-based pulmonary function tests (Finkelstein et al., 2000). He said that as the volume of patient data collected increases, it will be important to prioritize deviations (e.g., in blood pressure or glucose levels) and determine when clinical follow up is warranted. "We can't send everyone for appointments, and we can't alert doctors or patients all day long," he said. He suggested using data science and human–computer engineering principles to better optimize health monitoring technology use. For example, he described how personalized computational modeling was used to predict glucose levels in patients with diabetes based on their meals and their physiology. This information can be used to supplement glucose measurement in guiding patients' self-management. (Albers et al., 2017; Mamykina et al., 2016; Mamykina et al., 2017). He stressed that improved EHR systems will better support oncology care and help realize the vision of a learning health system.

Hripcsak predicted that a "major usability breakthrough" in EHRs is on the horizon. He suggested future EHRs for cancer care will be more patient focused, will facilitate earlier and more targeted interventions that are less toxic, and will also prioritize cancer prevention interventions. He suggested that the EHR could evolve into a "life record" that incorporates mobile computing, physiologic monitoring, and social media, for example, that will inform and advise patients and their care team. He elaborated that the EHR could contain baseline genomic information about a patient's tumor, periodic laboratory testing and imaging, and ongoing health monitoring from wearables, including the potential to detect and record environmental exposures (e.g., carcinogens, allergens, microbes, oxygen levels, meal composition).

Key Considerations for the Next Generation of EHRs

Many workshop speakers discussed opportunities for next-generation EHRs to improve patient care. Patel and Basch said EHRs are a tool to facilitate more patient-centered decision making for cancer care. Part of this is leveraging the EHR to better communicate with patients and develop a shared understanding of their health needs and the issues of greatest importance to them. Takvorian said the EHR can contribute to "amplifying the patient voice and the patient experience." Basch suggested creating incentives for EHR vendors to develop flexible EHR platforms and patient portals that will better enable practices to be patient centered. Robin Yabroff, scientific vice president of health services research at the American Cancer Society, said that EHR vendors need to engage patients to understand how they want to use the portal, especially when vendors make modifications or add new features to the patient portal.

Osterman said the next generation of EHRs could enable clinicians to think beyond managing an individual patient to managing populations of patients. For example, the EHR system could identify patients who might benefit from a newly approved treatment. He also highlighted the value of being able to access a new patient's medical records across health care systems and stressed the need for improved interoperability of EHRs and robust HIE. Basch raised the issue of the high cost of cancer treatment, and he noted that information about a patient's financial status or potential financial hardship could be entered into the EHR in order involve appropriate care team members to help patients with all aspects of their care (e.g., financial navigator, social worker).

Takvorian highlighted the critical importance of ensuring that all patients equally benefit from the opportunities afforded by next-generation EHRs. He said that EHRs have a potential role in promoting health equity in cancer care by, for example, countering implicit biases through more objective assessments and clinical decision-support recommendations. However, disparities could also be exacerbated by differences in patient ability to access or interact with their EHR or ancillary applications. He noted that Penn Medicine is reviewing its PRO-monitoring program to better understand observed disparities in reporting patterns, including which patients report and what information they report. Basch said that some patients with cancer in his health system were not receiving the COVID-19 vaccine because sign-up was initially only available via the patient portal. Once the health system became aware of this obstacle, health system staff used information in the EHR to identify patients who were not accessing the portal and reached out by telephone to schedule vaccine appointments. He said understanding which modes of communication a patient uses will help ensure that disparities are not unintentionally perpetuated due to missed communication. Hripcsak cautioned against making assumptions about which patients might be at a disadvantage as technologies evolve (e.g., those who are older or of lower economic means).

Workshop speakers also discussed opportunities to streamline EHRs by removing unnecessary elements. Hripcsak said that as new decision support rules are added, there should be a mechanism for the removal of obsolete rules. Takvorian suggested that, as patients have more access to their EHR and as billing practices evolve, EHRs will evolve away from inclusion of a lengthy, complex clinician note toward "meaningful notes that can promote a dialogue between patient and clinician." Hripcsak attributed some of the content and length of the clinical note to auditing requirements, explaining that clinicians have increasingly felt obligated to copy and paste laboratory or imaging results into the note to prove they had reviewed them. Addressing this issue is part of the AMIA 25x5 initiative, he said. Hripcsak and Osterman said that EHR vendors and professional societies both have roles in advancing the usability of EHRs.

To reduce documentation burdens on clinicians, Takvorian said there are opportunities to conduct pragmatic studies to assess questions about what aspects of the EHR work effectively and under what circumstances, and what aspects create or exacerbate problems. He called for publishing and disseminating the findings from these studies. Shulman reiterated that key patient data need to be readily accessible to clinicians and emphasized the need to focus on patient safety. Basch said there is a need to distinguish between what aspects of EHR systems are contributing to unnecessary clinician burden and the inherent challenges related to the complexities of cancer care.

Basch added that EHR developers need to understand that "contemporary cancer care is team-based care" and to develop systems that ensure that key information reaches the relevant team members so they can take the necessary actions. He said that the rigidity of the workflow of these systems sometimes results in team members receiving information or alerts that are not relevant to their role. Hripcsak said that all actions in the EHR have a cost, and the utility and cost of each action should be understood (e.g., the implications for patient care, health care team member satisfaction). Hripcsak stressed that adding a new functionality, such as an alert, is not free from burden. Shulman stressed that the implications of any action that increases clinician burden is amplified by the number of patients a clinician sees: A change to an EHR system that adds 5 minutes per patient could result in more than 1.5 hours of work each day for a clinician who sees 20 patients per day.

OPTIMIZING THE FUNCTIONALITY AND USABILITY OF EHRs IN ONCOLOGY CARE

A challenge for optimizing the functionally of EHRs for oncology care is that EHR systems have evolved to serve a range of competing uses and users, said Alexander Melamed, assistant professor in the Division of Gynecologic Oncology in the Department of Obstetrics and Gynecology at New York Presbyterian Hospital and Columbia University Medical Center. Many workshop speakers discussed opportunities to improve the functionality of EHRs in supporting care management, patient safety, and critical decision making; how an iterative human-centered design approach can be used to build EHR systems that better integrate into the clinical workflow and better meet the needs of patients across the cancer care continuum; and the importance of interoperability of systems.

Critical Decision Support

Many workshop speakers discussed the design and role of decision support tools that integrate clinical pathways within EHR systems to facilitate the delivery of evidence-based, safe, efficient, and high-value patient care.

Improving the Integration of Oncology Clinical Pathways in the EHR

Clinical pathways are care management tools to help clinicians and their patients select an evidence-based, cost-effective treatment approach that best meets a patient's clinical needs, social circumstances, and personal preferences, said Robin Zon, a community medical oncologist, immediate past president of Michiana Hematology Oncology, and co-chair of the American Society of Clinical Oncology (ASCO) Telehealth Expert Panel. She defined clinical pathways as a set of clinical decision support rules that integrate evidence regarding clinical effectiveness, potential risks for toxicity, and the cost of treatment in order to create optimal standard-of-care treatment recommendations for patients and reduce unnecessary variation in care.

Zon said the vision for integrating clinical pathways within an EHR system is

- to help ensure the patient has comprehensive, high-quality, cost-effective, patient-centered care across the entire continuum of cancer care;
- to serve as a platform for knowledge management and patient and clinician education about interventions; and
- to promote value-based care through the collection and analysis of pathway utilization data.

Zon highlighted several barriers to achieving this vision. First, there is inconsistent integration of oncology clinical pathways into EHR systems and within the clinical practice workflow. Lack of integration results in additional work for members of the health care team, interrupts daily tasks, may interfere with the clinician's ability to make patient care recommendations in real time, and may also result in delays of care. She shared her personal experience of having to enter a patient's staging data in the EHR, then exit the EHR and enter the same data elsewhere in order to navigate the recommended care pathway and search for potentially relevant clinical trials. Zon noted that the ASCO Task Force on Clinical Pathways[18] published criteria for evaluating clinical pathways and that these criteria discuss integration within the EHR and clinical workflow.

Costs of integrating clinical pathways into an EHR system can be prohibitive for an oncology practice group, said Zon, adding that clinicians are not currently reimbursed for pathway utilization or for the costs associated with clinical pathways integration within EHRs or updates. Costs also accrue when payers use

---

[18] See https://www.asco.org/news-initiatives/current-initiatives/cancer-care-initiatives/clinical-pathways (accessed September 7, 2022).

different clinical pathways, requiring administrative time to manage operational complexities, she said.

"Not all EHRs are created equal," Zon continued. Some practices have systems that are functional but are less common or older, and vendors only tend to develop clinical pathways that integrate with the most common EHR systems. While this is understandable from a business perspective, Zon said, it results in disparities in capabilities across practices, which could result in different outcomes for patients. She suggested that mandating EHR vendor compliance with existing and new EHR interoperability standards would encourage clinical pathway vendors and institutions to support increased functionality of EHR systems with embedded clinical pathways, while also minimizing resource utilization (financial, IT, administrative, training, etc.). She also suggested that payers provide incentives for clinical pathway integration and use, such as through value-based payment models that provide incentives for practices to procure and integrate current EHR and pathway technologies.

Zon said clinical pathways that are institutionally based (such as that developed by Kaiser, see below) can be monitored and kept up to date locally in response to new evidence and scientific knowledge. Some practices and systems purchase clinical pathway programs, and Zon has observed that vendors have been very responsive in making modifications quickly based on new knowledge. Zon said payer-facing clinical pathways can be more challenging to update, especially with regard to drug selection for a patient. If a clinical practice implements a pathway change, but the payer has not yet updated the pathway, the clinical practice might be penalized for not following their outdated pathway.

Improving Decision Support through Structured EHR Data

Mary Ichiuji, an oncologist at Kaiser Permanente (KP), and the national physician lead for the KP HealthConnect Oncology Beacon module, described the internal development and implementation of KP National Oncology Drug Treatment Pathways, an evidence-based EHR-integrated decision support tool that Ichiuji said enables the equitable delivery of cancer care to Kaiser Permanente members.

Kaiser Permanente serves 12.5 million members in eight regions of the United States, and its 305 oncologists order more than 60,000 treatment plans per year, said Ichiuji. In 2005, KP deployed the Epic Beacon oncology module, called HealthConnect, within its EHR. Ichiuji said Beacon is a computerized physician order entry system that enables "evidence-based, standardized, safe ordering and administration of cost-effective therapy across our organization." A multidisciplinary group meets weekly to maintain the library of nearly 1,200 protocols, and Ichiuji noted that KP does not require preauthorizations.

In 2018, KP began to develop internal oncology treatment pathways that would be fully integrated with its EHR through the Beacon module, Ichiuji said. The requirements for the decision support tool were defined as follows:

- Evidence-based
- Inclusion of information on efficacy, toxicity, and cost to organization
- Easy to use (3 additional clicks)
- Up to date (edited quarterly)
- Preferred vs. alternative options
- Emphasis on clinical trials
- Inclusion of palliative care/hospice
- Feedback
- Metrics

Ichiuji added that pathway development considers major compendia, relative efficacy, side effect profiles, and cost.

An initial clinical pathway draft was developed by regional subspecialty groups, and after a national subspecialty consensus process and approval by the governance group of interregional oncology chiefs, the clinical pathways were integrated into the KP clinical library and linked to the EHR through Beacon. Ichiuji said KP determined that the clinical pathways needed to be viewable from the EHR or the intranet, orderable from the patient chart, and utilize a minimal number of clicks to move from the chart to the clinical library and through the ordering process.

KP Oncology Pathways currently has 126 pathways covering 37 diseases. Pathways are updated routinely and can be modified quickly to address practice-changing information, such as severe drug shortages, the withdrawal of an indication for a particular drug, or discontinuation of a protocol. There is a link for users to provide feedback as well as a link to return to the EHR to complete the order if a pathway is not available. Pathways display preferred and alternative treatment protocols; they also contain links to relevant clinical trials websites, have the ability to email the relevant subspecialty group, and include a "hover-to-discover" feature that pops up additional information related to a pathway element, such as "clinical pearls" about dosing of a drug or therapy and links to references.

In 2021, KP began measuring regional-, medical center-, and clinician-level pathway usage, and analyses have found that pathway usage is increasing monthly in all regions, Ichiuji said. Data are also being collected regarding which treatment pathway was used (preferred, alternative, off-pathway) to inform future care choices. Kaiser Permanente is now working to build a comprehensive cancer pathway to support patients across the continuum of cancer care, which Ichiuji said will include decision support and population health tools for risk stratification, screening and automated outreach, diagnosis, molecular genomics, treatment, symptom management, self-care and psychosocial support, survivorship surveillance, and healthy-lifestyle engagement. She added that patient voices are incorporated into this process.

Creating an Efficient EHR Workspace that Presents Critical Data to Oncology Clinicians

Shilo Anders, a research associate professor in the department of anesthesiology, biomedical informatics, and computer science at Vanderbilt University and member of the Center for Research and Innovation in System Safety (CRISS), said that current EHRs are generally not ideal workspaces, and safety is a concern when systems are stretched beyond their original design or intent, particularly in the context of health care.

One approach to improving the functionality of the EHR for critical decision making is to capture nonroutine events in the EHR, including those that occur outside of the hospital system, Anders said. A nonroutine event is one that results in a deviation from the patient's optimal care path, which increases their risk for adverse outcomes. Over the past two decades, CRISS has been studying these deviations to understand if there are underlying safety issues that can be addressed, or interventions to adopt, to improve the delivery of high-quality care.

Anders shared several examples of nonroutine events that patients with cancer have experienced. Some events relate to equipment or technology, such as when a patient alerted the care team that his feeding tube was left unclamped after being adjusted, but his concern was not addressed, resulting in leakage. Another event occurred when a patient became increasingly distraught and potentially suicidal while experiencing severe treatment side effects. Although he reported his distress to his clinicians via the patient portal, his concerns were not discussed until he had an appointment with his clinicians. In another case, a patient experienced increasing, uncontrolled pain over a weekend and had forgotten that they had pain medication they could take.

A study by CRISS of 106 nonroutine events found that 86 percent occurred at home, and the majority were associated with a patient's treatment (38 percent associated with chemotherapy, 32 percent with radiation therapy, 7 percent with surgery) (unpublished data). Anders noted that less than half of these nonroutine events were reported to the care team by the patient. Capturing nonroutine events could improve the design of the EHR workspace to more readily present critical safety and care information to the oncology care team that is both intelligible and actionable, she said.

Applying a Human-Centered Design Approach to Improving EHR Systems

Many workshop speakers discussed applying a human-centered design approach to improving EHR systems (Figure 5). Anders said there is often a disconnect between what is thought about how people use a system or technology and how they actually use it. EHR systems were developed based on how their use was imagined, which was drawn from experiences at static points in time. However, EHRs are implemented in a system that is dynamic and stochastic. Human-centered design is an iterative approach that works directly with end users to understand how they interact with the system to accomplish tasks and achieve goals. "Normal work is not well behaved, especially in the clinical environment," she said. Human-centered design provides "opportunities to more closely align the fit of the EHR to the cancer care system," by asking questions about how clinicians and patients use the EHR and what their needs are. For example, what is the best way to get new information to clinicians? How should nonroutine events and other PRO data be visualized? Would including ML outputs in the EHR contribute to diagnostic accuracy or add too much complexity and confusion?

The Interface between Electronic Systems and Humans

Elizabeth Mynatt, dean of the Khoury College of Computer Sciences at Northeastern University, discussed MyPath, a personalized, adaptive mobile tool

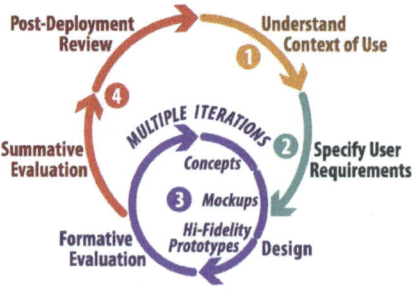

FIGURE 5 Human-centered approach to EHR design.
SOURCE: Anders presentation, February 28, 2022. Copyright, 2014. Weinger, Beebe, Center for Research and Innovation in Systems Safety, and Vanderbilt University Medical Center. All rights reserved.

to support patients across their cancer care continuum.[19] Mynatt said the intent was to create "an information ecosystem that could surround and center on the patient," not only providing medical information but also taking into account their daily responsibilities, personal experiences, SDOH, and other factors.

The process of creating the technology began with understanding the role and practices of navigators who worked with patients with breast cancer in rural northwest Georgia. Mynatt and colleagues then developed a framework outlining a patient's health care responsibilities (e.g., treatment adherence, managing side effects), personal challenges they face when receiving cancer treatment, and the impact of cancer on their daily life (Table 1) (see Hayes et al., 2008; Jacobs et al., 2014, 2017).

The technology was designed to be holistic and personalized, pulling information from the EHR and adding information about the patient that might affect their experience with cancer care (e.g., socioeconomic status, daily responsibilities). Mynatt said it is also adaptive, customizing content based on the patient's evolving goals, needs, and priorities. Key features of the technology are an open, customizable platform; integration into the health system; and a simple artificial intelligence (AI) system to index vetted resources against their diagnosis, treatment plan, and PROs. In addition to the patient information outputs, there are metrics and usage data (Jacobs et al., 2018, 2019).

The prototype tool was a mobile device and Mynatt said, ideally, it would be an app. She showed the MyPath patient interface, which she said is a "one-stop shop" for information about the patient's specific cancer, treatments, social supports, health and well-being, and emotional support. There are personalized resources and suggestions for handling day-to-day matters (e.g., financial concerns, transportation, childcare, diet, talking to the doctor about side effects). There is also a survey, which users are prompted to complete regularly, to inform the personalization of the content.

Mynatt highlighted the importance of presenting timely, relevant information that engages patients over the long term, not just immediately after diagnosis, and promotes their confidence in engaging with the care team. In addition, the information collected from patients via the tool helps with care coordination, and she noted that "patients would tell the system things that they would not tell their physician." Mynatt also mentioned that patients have reported getting conflicting guidance from different specialty clinicians (e.g., the oncologist versus the endocrinologist they see for their diabetes) and want to know, "Which is right?" She suggested that patients should be able to flag such conflicts in the EHR so they can be addressed. Finally, Mynatt suggested that oncology clinical pathways and the patient's experiences across the cancer care continuum could

---

[19] Mynatt stated that her presentation was drawn largely from the dissertation work of her former student, Maia Jacobs, while at the Georgia Institute of Technology.

TABLE 1 Framework for a Patient's Health Care Responsibilities and Challenges and Their Impact on Daily Life

	Responsibilities	**Challenges**	**Personal Journey**
	Patient work Health tasks placed on patient	Barriers to care	The effects of cancer on one's personal, daily life
Screening and Diagnosis	Communicating the disease to others	Information gaps Emotional impacts Dealing with others' reactions	Attitude changes Major life events
Information Seeking	Information filtering and organization Clinical decisions Preparation	Overwhelming amount of information Understanding treatment options	Coping strategies
Acute Care and Treatment	Symptom management Support management Compliance Managing clinical transitions Financial management	Inability to work Transportation Lack of support Reluctance to ask for help Unexpected complications	Relationship changes Responsibilities of daily life Social behavior changes Loss of independence Asserting control Health milestones
No Evidence of Disease	Continued monitoring Giving back to the community Health behavior changes	Worry about recurrence	Survivor identity Return to normal

SOURCE: Mynatt presentation, February 28, 2022, reprinted from Jacobs et al., 2017.

inform each other. Although information from clinical pathways is used to support the patient's care, she proposed that information from the patient experience be better integrated and leveraged to refine the decision support tools within clinical pathways.

Systems Engineering for EHR Design in Oncology Care

Pascale Carayon, professor emerita in the department of industrial and systems engineering at the University of Wisconsin–Madison and founding director of the Wisconsin Institute for Healthcare Systems Engineering, described the Systems Engineering Initiative for Patient Safety (SEIPS) 3.0 model for patient care, a sociotechnical systems approach to improving patient safety and other outcomes (Carayon et al., 2020). Patients with cancer interact with multiple elements of work systems as they receive care across space and time (Figure 6). The care team functions within the context of their physical environment, organizational conditions, tasks, and tools and technologies (e.g., EHRs). The model focuses on how to design work systems to promote patient safety and achieve other desired outcomes for patients, caregivers, clinicians, and health care organizations. Feedback loops in the model facilitate continuous learning, adaptation, and improvement of the work systems.

Carayon also discussed examples of applying human-centered design to improve the safety and functionality of tools and technologies. These included redesigning the placement of products in the medication drawer of a code cart to improve the safety and efficiency of drug administration (Rousek and Hallbeck, 2011), and redesigning the EHR interface used by clinicians in the intensive care unit for more efficient and clear presentation of critical data to support decision making (Pickering et al., 2010).

Human-centered design of tools and technologies draws on the principles and methods of the scientific discipline of human factors and ergonomics, including usability heuristics and usability evaluation, Carayon said (see Kortum, 2016). It is a structured approach to designing technologies that support work. Carayon reiterated the points by Anders that user-centered or human-centered design of the EHR requires an understanding of the actual work that clinicians, patients, and other users do, not what it is thought that they do. As such, participation of the health care team—including patients—is essential to the design process. Carayon noted that participants bring multiple perspectives, and it is important to resolve conflicts and develop a common ground. Learning through feedback loops is also needed to support a continuous design and implementation process (Carayon and Salwei, 2021).

User-centered EHR technologies also need to fit the workflow (i.e., inte-

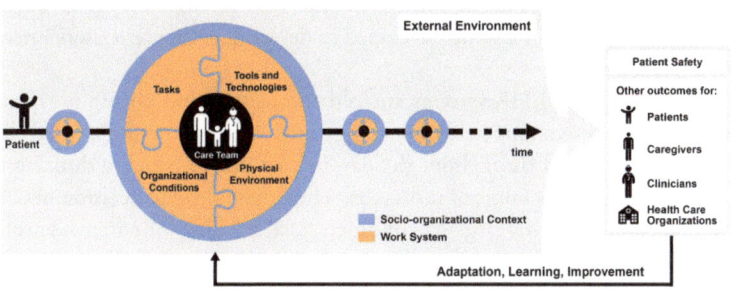

FIGURE 6 Systems Engineering Initiative for Patient Safety (SEIPS) 3.0 model of patient care.
SOURCE: Carayon presentation, February 28, 2022, reprinted from Carayon et al. (2020).

grate with the other elements of the work system). Carayon noted that poorly designed EHR technologies and interfaces can negatively affect patient–clinician communication and have been found to contribute to burnout and stress for both clinicians and patients (Gajra et al., 2020; Haider et al., 2018; Lafferty et al., 2021; Tetzlaff et al., 2022). Key design considerations include how the technology supports the task and how it fits with the temporal flow and the physical environment of the tasks and with other technologies.

Carayon called for EHR technologies to be designed to support patients across the entire cancer care continuum, taking into consideration evolving work systems and fluid care teams—who are situated across time, space, and organizations—and incorporating interfaces that support care coordination (Lichtner and Baysari, 2021; Lichtner et al., 2020).

EHR Vendor Perspective on EHR Design

Jenna Date shared her perspective as the chief experience officer for health care solutions at Allscripts Hospital and Health Systems, a vendor of health care IT solutions, including EHR systems. The focus of her work at Allscripts is human-centered design, and she described a recent project where Allscripts staff spent time observing clinicians at work at five oncology clinics across three sites. The practices varied in size, from a practice that included one oncologist and an assistant to large practices that included health professional education and training programs. The goal, she said, was to use retrospective techniques and contextual inquiry to obtain a holistic impression of "a day in the life of an oncologist."

Date described a technique called personas to model user needs. Personas are fictional characterizations of the users of a technology that are designed based on discussions with actual users. For example, she said they developed personas to model what acute care hospitalists needed to accomplish using a new mobile technology during the 30 seconds to 3 minutes they had between patients. User maps can also be developed to depict how different users interact with a technology.

Date said many EHR systems are "old and brittle" and not up to the task of supporting the dynamic field of oncology care. Allscripts staff observed clinicians running behind throughout the day, in part due to issues with using the EHR technology for a range of tasks (e.g., scheduling, dosing, decision making, organizing and executing large sets of orders, task tracking for patients enrolled in clinical trials, regulatory compliance, administrative tasks). Date said they also found that many clinicians are still keeping paper records alongside their EHR system.

Allscripts is working to co-create the EHR experience with clinicians and patients so that EHR products fit better into their daily lives, not just into the workflow, Date said. Their focus is on simplicity and getting back to basic tasks, she said, using AI to reduce regulatory and administrative "noise" in the EHR so clinicians can focus on patient care.

Integration and Interoperability to Improve EHR Functionality and Support a Learning Health Care System

Zon, Ichiuji, Mynatt, and others emphasized the need for interoperability of systems. "It seems like we're always working for the EHR and the pathway," Zon said. "The EHR and pathway need to be working for us." She said the lack of interoperability is a key underlying factor that negatively affects EHR functionality and usability and frustrates both clinicians and patients. She called for EHR systems be held to interoperability standards, adding that change is unlikely to happen without advocacy for new policies or mandates.

Bradley Malin, professor of biomedical informatics, biostatistics, and computer science at Vanderbilt University, asked speakers to consider where the EHR system ends, and other systems begin, and to what extent data need to be formalized versus letting some information remain "a little bit soft and squishy to allow for flexibility." Date said that technology could help manage the interface of "soft and squishy" and formalized information. Artificial intelligence and digital assistants could be deployed to help clinicians make smarter decisions based on their interactions with the patient. The question is whether and how such information is preserved—that is, does it remain as a verbal discussion between the patient and clinician, or does it need to be recorded or formalized? She added that many clinicians have expressed a desire for better ways to connect with patients as well as concern that the clinical note is not typically written in a patient-centered manner because it is intended for many different audiences, including other clinicians, auditors, payers, and regulators.

Zon pointed out that clinical pathways make standard-of-care recommendations based on high-level evidence, but they can be rigid, making it difficult to apply the guidance to personalized, shared decision making with a patient. She said that the developers of clinical pathways and EHR systems need to collaborate better to foster a learning health care system, collecting and analyzing data about pathway use, including data about when clinicians deviate from pathways to personalize care.

Mynatt said some information, such as certain PROs, can help to guide clinical decision making, but this type of information also has value outside the EHR. For example, cancer care navigators can use this information to identify community needs. Basch noted that approaches for third-party applications to connect with ease to EHRs would enable innovation in data collection, communication, and information portability.

IMPROVING EHR DATA COLLECTION TO SUPPORT CLINICAL CARE, QUALITY AND VALUE, AND RESEARCH

Many workshop speakers discussed opportunities to improve how EHR data are collected, documented, and shared to better support cancer care decision making, usability of data for research, and payer efforts to ensure care quality and value.

Improving Data Collection and Display to Support Clinical Decision Making

Oncology clinicians sift through the EHR to identify the critical data elements they need to assess, diagnose, and care for patients with cancer, said Tufia Haddad, associate professor of oncology at the Mayo Clinic College of Medicine and Science, and medical director of Care Anyplace at the Mayo Clinic Center for Digital Health. For example, as a breast oncologist, critical data elements she collects include patient attributes, such as age and menopause status; tumor-related attributes, such as germline mutations, TNM staging,[20] tumor grade, and relevant biomarkers; as well as a patient's past and current cancer treatments.

Although clinicians use information in the EHR, Haddad noted that clinical decision making remains a labor-intensive process in which clinicians primarily rely on their experience and content knowledge to make patient care decisions. She observed that some clinicians do not routinely access clinical decision support tools and resources, such as treatment guidelines or clinical pathways. However, she stressed that the volume and complexity of the data potentially available to guide decision making is ever increasing, so individual clinicians cannot possibly keep up to date on the advances in oncology care. "This model for clinical decision making simply is not sustainable," Haddad said.

Haddad called for changing how data are collected, organized, and labeled in the EHR to help alleviate the cognitive burden on the clinical care team, especially as the volume of information increases. She also suggested that clinicians increase the use of evidence-based guidelines to counter clinician biases and promote equitable cancer care.

Haddad said that standardized definitions of critical data elements and standardized templates for diagnostic reports and treatment plans are needed, with PROs systematically captured in the EHR. Critical data elements need

---

[20] TNM staging is a system used to describe the amount and spread of cancer in a patient's body. T describes the size of the tumor and any spread of cancer into nearby tissue; N describes spread of cancer to nearby lymph nodes; and M describes metastasis (spread of cancer to other parts of the body). See https://www.cancer.gov/about-cancer/diagnosis-staging/staging (accessed August 30, 2022).

to be labeled as such, and she said these data could be entered in a structured format or could be abstracted and interpreted from unstructured clinical notes and captured in the EHR using NLP and ML models. Haddad described how a synopsis of critical data elements could then be matched with patient-specific care recommendations, practice guidelines, and clinical trial opportunities "in one click" at the point of care. This information could then drive the selection of treatment plans and order sets, the collection of PROs, and smart appointment scheduling (e.g., duration and resources tailored to individual patient needs). It could also be used to automate the population of key documents such the patient's medical history, oncology history, and problem list, and share clinical information for downstream tasks (e.g., coding, billing, prior authorizations). This would enable clinicians to spend less time in front of the screen and more time in direct patient care, Haddad said.

Haddad added that curating these critical data elements in a robust data analytics infrastructure could facilitate population-based cancer surveillance activities in near real time, with the ability to update information for a given patient longitudinally. These registries could also be used for other purposes, including quality reporting, identifying future priorities for clinical research, and supporting retrospective research.

Standardizing how clinical data are documented in the EHR facilitates sharing information about the patient and better enables the development, validation, and training of NLP and ML algorithms and models, Haddad said. She emphasized that large data sets from diverse patient populations are needed to ensure that models are inclusive. It is also necessary to show reproducibility of these models across different health care organizations and patient populations.

Monica Bertagnolli, professor of surgery at Harvard Medical School and chief of the Division of Surgical Oncology at Brigham and Women's Hospital and the Dana-Farber Cancer Institute, also emphasized the need for structured, computable data that can be readily aggregated and shared at scale in order to support a learning health care system. She concurred with others that aggregated EHR data are often incomplete because many clinicians are still recording critical data elements in an unstructured, text-based format in the clinical note. "The mantra of efficient data use is collect it once, use it many times," Bertagnolli said. However, she noted that duplicative data entry persists, which is both ineffective and can introduce errors. She stressed that entering data in a standardized format facilitates interoperability and the use of these data for many purposes (e.g., registry reporting, prior authorization, quality reporting, matching patients with potential clinical trials, conducting clinical trials).

Bertagnolli also highlighted the mCODE initiative (previously discussed by Osterman), which is defining standardized oncology clinical data elements across six key domains. She said that data standards have to serve the needs of oncologists and patients if they are to succeed. The mCODE initiative is working with EHR vendors to develop health records with standard data elements to facilitate interoperability. The CodeX community[21] is driving the adoption of mCODE standards and developing tools that utilize mCODE standardized data. Bertagnolli also noted that another group called Gravity[22] is focused on developing standards to capture SDOH data.

Barry Russo, chief executive officer at The Center for Cancer and Blood Disorders, discussed EHR interoperability challenges within his community oncology practice. The Center has 54 clinicians across 14 locations and currently operates three different EHR systems. The practice also has a clinical pathway system; a patient portal; triage, risk stratification, and clinical trial management systems; and work is underway to develop a PRO reporting system. He said there are many connectivity and interoperability challenges across the components of these internal practice systems, as well as with external EHR systems and applications at the nearly 40 hospitals in the Dallas–Fort Worth area where Center physicians practice. Although the practice is working to collect and record structured data using both NLP and staff data abstraction, the extracted data are not as clean as expected, contributing to challenges in assembling cohorts of patients, he said.

Russo said the Center created a "data lake," an external data center where disparate pieces of data from across these many data streams are aggregated into usable data sets that can then be accessed for continuous quality improvement projects. He noted that this process is time consuming and involves a lot of manual work by many analysts.

While the practice is addressing interoperability of systems and standardization of data broadly, Russo reported that clinicians are most concerned about the number of "clicks" needed to complete patient data entry and other clinical tasks in the course of caring for 25 to 30 patients each day. "My physicians could tell you how many clicks each section of the [EHR] requires," he said. He reiterated the point by Zon and others that EHR systems need to work for clinicians, instead of clinicians feeling like they work for the EHR.

Opportunities to Improve the Usability of EHRs for Research Purposes

Jeremy Warner, adjunct associate professor of medicine at Vanderbilt University, discussed challenges and opportunities associated with using EHRs for research purposes. The structured data elements in the EHR include the International Classification of Disease (ICD) codes. Warner pointed out that ICD codes support the billing of services rendered but do not necessarily indi-

---

[21] See https://confluence.hl7.org/display/COD/CodeX+Home (accessed August 30, 2022).

[22] See https://www.hl7.org/gravity/ (accessed August 30, 2022).

cate a confirmed diagnosis. For example, the code U07.1 was created in 2020 to identify laboratory-confirmed SARS-CoV-2, but he said this code has been used to justify billing for diagnostic workups for patients with suspected infection (a.k.a. presumptive COVID-19), whether or not the patient was ultimately diagnosed with SARS-CoV-2 infection. To address this, the code U07.2, for "COVID-19, virus not identified" was introduced, but Warner said it was not adopted in the United States and is not recorded in EHRs. Further, there is currently no ICD code for when COVID-19 was suspected but a different illness was confirmed.

Another challenge of using EHRs to conduct meaningful research is disconnected systems of clinical care and the poor interoperability of these systems. A patient with cancer often receives care across many years, within different health care systems, and in different geographic settings, Warner said. His research has also shown that laboratory values and patient demographic data are inconsistently represented across EHRs, even within the same EHR vendor system (Bernstam et al., 2022). Further, knowing the provenance of data (e.g., who ordered a test, interpreted a test, etc.) is important, but Warner said this information can be lost when data are aggregated.

Warner also observed that there is a "tension between narrative and structured text in the EHR" and suggested that there will continue to be a need for narrative description in the EHR. He described clinical narrative as "one of the most complex domains of human written discourse" and said that cutting-edge ML and AI techniques are being developed to extract and standardize information from EHRs.

Warner said that an evolved EHR ecosystem could present improved opportunities for research through the integration of genomic and other molecular information. "Precision oncology can't happen without marrying the phenome and the genome, and the EHR is the logical place for this to happen," Warner said. He also suggested empowering patients to use their own data to make discoveries about themselves and to share their findings with their clinical team and the research commons.

Warner referred participants to the Informatics Technology for Cancer Research program at the NCI for more information about ongoing research to address informatics needs across the cancer continuum.[23]

Opportunities to Improve EHR Data Collection to Support High-Quality Care and Value

Payers need actionable and comprehensive data to achieve their goal of enhancing value in the delivery of health care, said Reed Tuckson, cofounder of

---

[23] See https://itcr.cancer.gov (accessed May 18, 2022).

the Black Coalition Against COVID and managing director of Tuckson Health Connections, LLC. These data can be collected as part of clinical research or captured during the delivery of clinical care. Tuckson said payers use data to help achieve a wide range of quality and value objectives. He said there is payer interest in supporting clinician and patient decision making; closing gaps in care; reducing waste; addressing increasing costs; bringing innovations more quickly to patients; advancing the evidence base for care delivery; personalizing patient care based on evolving knowledge; controlling capital expenditures related to the acquisition, maintenance, and use of data systems and assets; ensuring patient privacy; addressing the issue of data ownership; and fostering trust in the patient–clinician relationship.

Tuckson also suggested that payers could offer incentives to promote patient and clinician involvement in clinical trials as well as data collection and sharing across the continuum of care. Further, he said that incentives could be offered to payers for active participation in clinical research (e.g., awarding plans extra points toward their annual performance or "star" ratings). He noted there are also lessons to be learned from the implementation and use of the National Patient-Centered Clinical Research Network Distributed Data Network.[24]

Suggestions to Improve Data Collection and Promote Data Sharing

Several workshop speakers discussed how to improve data collection at the point of care and promote greater usability of EHR technology in clinical practice. Warner suggested that health professional education and training programs prioritize best practices for clinical documentation and emphasize the importance of entering structured data where possible.

To receive buy-in from clinical practices, Haddad suggested focusing less on the technologies themselves and more on how using them could help solve some of the challenges clinicians and oncology practices are facing (e.g., reducing administrative and cognitive burdens, keeping up to date with the rapid advancement of medical knowledge, facilitating clinical trial enrollment, addressing disparities in health care). She also suggested collaborating with experts in human-centered design and engineering—alongside technology vendors—to retool clinical workflows to meet user needs.

Haddad said policies are needed to support the interoperability of the EHRs and facilitate data sharing. Bertagnolli agreed and said that participants in the research and health care enterprises have an obligation to share patient data, with approval from the patient. She stressed that health data belong to patients and, in her experience, "patients want us to appropriately share the data and use it to gain

---

[24] See https://pcornet.org/ (accessed September 7, 2022).

new knowledge." She observed that although data sharing policies are in place, systems often have a range of reasons for why they are unwilling to share.

Tuckson suggested there is a need to revisit the HIPAA Privacy Rule because, as it is currently implemented, it can impede data sharing and the conduct of health research (IOM, 2009). Warner agreed and said that the Privacy Rule is "more of an impediment to data sharing than it is protection for patients." He suggested patients could be asked if they are willing to share their data for specified purposes beyond providing them with care (e.g., academic research or commercial research and development).

Russo proposed creating a national HIE to generate real-world datasets that clinicians could use to inform care decisions for their patients. He suggested the effort be funded in part by payers, who would benefit from access to this information, and that participation by clinicians could be incentivized by linking it to reimbursement.

FEDERAL AGENCIES AS PARTNERS IN DRIVING EHR INNOVATION

Speakers representing the White House Office of Science and Technology Policy (OSTP), the NCI, the Centers for Disease Control and Prevention (CDC), the FDA, the Office of the National Coordinator for Health Information Technology (ONC), and CMS discussed the role of federal partners in helping to advance the functionality and usability of EHRs for cancer care, surveillance, and research.

OSTP: The Role of Science and Technology Policy in Advancing EHRs

The federal government is a producer and a consumer of innovation, and also a benefactor and a beneficiary of the products of innovation, said Bich-Thuy (Twee) Sim, assistant director of Transformative Medicine and Health Innovation at OSTP and senior medical advisor and lead of infectious diseases in the Defense Health Agency at the Department of Defense. The government serves as a partner and collaborator and supports sustainability through standards and regulatory processes, she said.

OSTP is uniquely positioned to serve as a convening body for participants from the federal sector, as well as from the private, academic, and public sectors, said Sim. She discussed some of the ongoing initiatives of the new OSTP Health and Life Sciences division, including biopreparedness (which includes pandemic preparedness); health systems and health equity, which Sim said includes EHRs; accelerating innovation, especially in the area of cancer; biomanufacturing; agriculture (as it relates to nutrition); and the life sciences research community (e.g., more inclusive doctoral education opportunities). The division is actively involved in a broad range of topics, including SDOH, AI and ML, biases in health care, and health communications.

Sim said the Biden Administration announced on February 2, 2022, a "reignition" of the Cancer Moonshot [25] noting that the goals are "to reduce the death rate from cancer by at least 50 percent over the next 25 years and to improve the experience of people and their families living with and surviving cancer and, by doing these and more, hope to end cancer as we know it today."[26] President Biden has also "proposed one of the largest science and technology budget increases in history," Sim said.

The NCI: Using EHR Data for Cancer Surveillance

Lynne Penberthy, associate director for the Surveillance Research Program in the Division of Cancer Control and Population Sciences at the NCI, explained that under state public health recording laws, central cancer registries are legally authorized to access health records. Because much of the relevant data for cancer surveillance are in unstructured text formats in EHRs, surveillance currently requires manual review, annotation, and extraction of data, which Penberthy said is estimated to require more than 60,000 person-hours per year. Penberthy said this is unsustainable, especially given the increasing volume of data needed for cancer surveillance (e.g., longitudinal treatment history, genomic characterization of tumors). In addition, the NCI Surveillance, Epidemiology, and End Results (SEER) Program[27] is moving toward near real-time reporting of incidence data, which also makes manual data extraction impractical. There is also inconsistent capture in EHRs of the data needed for surveillance, because patients often receive care at several different facilities. She discussed two targeted solutions the NCI is developing to address these challenges to illustrate how a federal agency can support the advancement of EHRs for cancer surveillance.

Penberthy first discussed how the NCI is working with the Department of Energy to develop algorithms for automated extraction of key structured data from unstructured EHR text using deep learning and NLP. She described how they are targeting pathology and radiology reports because they contain key tumor characterization data needed for surveillance, specifically, tumor site, histology, laterality, and behavior. Penberthy noted that there are many challenges. For example, there is inconsistent content across the unstructured text entered by thousands of pathologists across the United States, and there are more than

---

[25] The 21st Century Cures Act, passed in 2016, authorized $1.8 billion in funding over seven years to support cancer research and the "Cancer Moonshot" initiative.

[26] See https://www.whitehouse.gov/briefing-room/statements-releases/2022/02/02/fact-sheet-president-biden-reignites-cancer-moonshot-to-end-cancer-as-we-know-it/

[27] See https://seer.cancer.gov/ (accessed September 1, 2022).

500 histology categories and over 100 cancer site classifications. There is also limited data available for algorithm development, especially for rare tumors and histologies.

Manually extracted data from seven registries are being used to train the algorithm and to develop an application programming interface (API)[28] for processing unstructured pathology reports, Penberthy said. The process involves iterative testing, development, and retraining of the algorithm. An uncertainty quantification process was developed that identifies reports with less than 97 percent accuracy and flags them for human review.

Thus far, the API has been implemented into the production workflow of 11 SEER registries, facilitating automatic and highly accurate processing of approximately 25 percent of the more than four million pathology reports the NCI receives annually, Penberthy said. The automated process is 18,000 times faster than human extraction of the data, she said, saving more than 11,500 hours of labor. The workflow is being leveraged to facilitate iterative improvement of the algorithm (e.g., via human review of random samples of auto-coded reports) and to train personnel to improve the consistency of manual reports. Penberthy said the API for pathology reports is also being adapted to process radiology reports.

The NCI is also creating data linkages to external organizations to leverage their source data for surveillance. For example, Penberthy said that SEER has established data linkages to Walgreens, CVS, and RiteAid pharmacies to provide information on oral drugs used for cancer treatment. Information on these drugs "is not routinely available to hospital registries through their EHRs," said Penberthy. One challenge to this approach is the variable and inconsistent insurance coverage of prescription drugs in the United States. Also, some cancer drugs are only provided by designated pharmacies, which, she noted, can change annually. The NCI is testing and implementing several solutions to address the gaps and reduce the biases that this could introduce into the data.

In the second use case, the NCI is creating linkages with selected genomic pathology laboratories that can provide comprehensive data for all patients receiving a particular genetic test (e.g., Oncotype DX 21 gene assay for breast cancer, Oncotype and Decipher multigene panels for prostate cancer, DecisionDX multigene panel for melanoma). A challenge for this approach is that the genomic pathology laboratories often only collect name, date of birth, and address, which can impede matching if a patient moves and their address at the time of testing does not match the address entered in the registry at initial diagnosis. To better adjudicate uncertain matches, Penberthy said that the SEER

---

[28] An API is a "set of definitions and protocols for building and integrating application software." https://www.redhat.com/en/topics/api/what-are-application-programming-interfaces (accessed September 1, 2022).

program now obtains longitudinal address information through Lexis Nexis searches and through manual reviews.

The CDC: Leveraging EHRs for Public Health Planning and Research

Lisa Richardson, director of the Division of Cancer Prevention and Control at the CDC, discussed how the CDC is using data from EHRs for public health planning and research. The National Program of Cancer Registries, authorized by Congress in 1992 and administered by the CDC, collects data from 50 State Central Cancer Registries (Figure 7). However, even in the era of EHRs, it remains challenging for cancer registrars to find the necessary information in a patient's record, Richardson said. She said the CDC and the College of American Pathologists developed an electronic cancer checklist for each major cancer type, which facilitates standardized documentation, reporting, and transmission of structured data by pathologists.

The CDC is also working to facilitate better communication and collaboration among health care systems and public health institutions. Richardson said the CDC is helping to build capacity for reporting via a cloud platform of the Association of Public Health Laboratories (APHL) Informatics Messaging Services (AIMS) that provides data sharing and processing services. She noted that 90 percent of State Central Cancer Registries are now able to receive pathology reports from APHL's AIMS cloud platform. Richardson noted that this information is critical for comprehensive cancer control planning, which she said requires timely and accurate data.

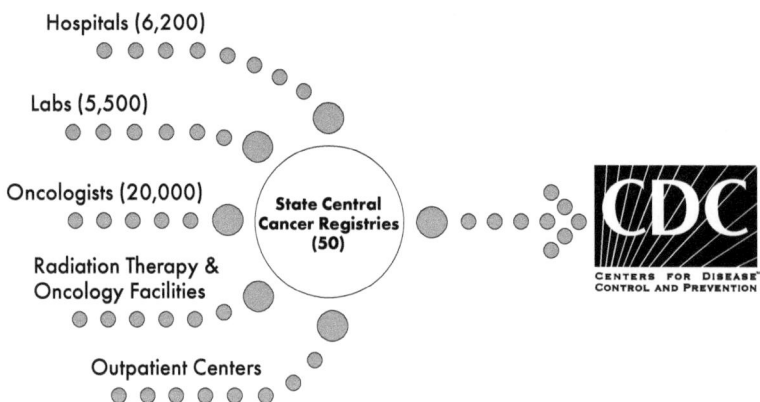

FIGURE 7 Flow of data to the CDC National Program of Cancer Registries.
SOURCE: Richardson presentation, March 1, 2022.

With funding from the Patient-Centered Outcomes Research Trust Fund, the CDC is studying how cloud computing could make EHR data more readily available for research and public health purposes. She outlined the vision for electronic case reporting of patient data using the cloud. After a patient is diagnosed with a reportable condition (such as cancer), a clinician would enter the information into the EHR, which would automatically trigger the creation and validation of a case report that is then sent to the relevant public health agencies. Public health agencies would receive the data in real time and respond to the clinician, and state and local health departments would take appropriate public health action (e.g., contact tracing, cancer control planning).

EHR systems can also be used to identify individuals who have missed cancer screenings or follow-up appointments, Richardson said, noting the rates of routine screenings for common cancers declined significantly during the height of the COVID-19 pandemic and are still below pre-pandemic levels.[29] Additionally, she cited a recent study that found 60 percent of women diagnosed with cervical cancer had never been screened, and two-thirds of women who had an abnormal screening result did not receive appropriate follow-up (Benard et al., 2021).

Richardson said that patients who receive care in safety-net settings face a myriad of barriers to obtaining cancer screening and follow-up care (e.g., safety-net settings may have insufficient staffing, limited health IT infrastructure, inadequate access to specialty care, and administrative challenges), which exacerbates health inequities. To promote equitable access to evidence-based cervical cancer screening, the CDC is working with MITRE Health to develop a clinical decision support tool that converts cervical cancer screening guidelines into a computable format. Based on the embedded guidelines, the tool will identify patients who are due for screening, send a reminder to the clinician, and link to the guidelines for follow-up care. Richardson emphasized that the goal is to integrate these capabilities without increasing the burden on clinicians.

The FDA: Using EHR Data to Generate Evidence for Oncology Product Development

The FDA reviews data from a range of sources when making science-based regulatory decisions about the efficacy and safety of new drug and biologic therapies, said Paul Kluetz, deputy director of the Oncology Center of Excellence at the FDA. To be confident in its conclusions about the risks and benefits of new treatments, the FDA needs evidence of causality (i.e., data

---

[29] See https://cancerletter.com/real-world-evidence/20210917_1/ (accessed May 18, 2022).

showing that an observed treatment benefit is due to the intervention and not a confounding influence). Randomized controlled trials have long been the key source of this evidence; however, the 21st Century Cures Act directed the FDA to create a framework to evaluate the use of real-world evidence in its decision making.[30]

Kluetz said there is a "critical distinction" between real-world data and real-word evidence. Real-world evidence is "the clinical evidence about the usage and potential benefits or risks of a medical product derived from real-world data." Real-world data are "data relating to patient health status and/or the delivery of health care routinely collected from a variety of sources." EHRs are one source of real-world data.

Although real-world data sources have been used primarily for nonrandomized, retrospective, observational studies, Kluetz said that EHR data can be leveraged for prospective randomized controlled trials, decentralized trials, and pragmatic trials as well. There are challenges for using EHR data to generate evidence of treatment benefit for investigational oncology products, Kluetz noted. For example, there is a lack of randomization, data are often unstructured and require curation, tumor-based endpoints are generally not recorded in the EHR, and movement of patients through different EHR systems can affect data quality and the completeness of data capture on treatment and outcomes.

A variety of FDA initiatives are underway to advance the utility of real-world data—including EHR data—to provide evidence suitable for regulatory decision making. Kluetz said the Oncology Center of Excellence has formed an oncology-specific Real-World Evidence program[31] that includes cross-FDA collaboration to develop consistent terminology and several external collaborations to improve source data (e.g., with mCODE,[32] ASH Collaborative[33]), better characterize real world data submissions (e.g., with Reagan-Udall Foundation Oncology QCARD project[34]), and develop real-world endpoints (e.g., with Friends of Cancer Research[35]).

---

[30] See https://www.fda.gov/science-research/science-and-research-special-topics/real-world-evidence (accessed September 1, 2022).

[31] See https://www.fda.gov/science-research/science-and-research-special-topics/real-world-evidence and https://www.fda.gov/about-fda/oncology-center-excellence/oncology-real-world-evidence-program (accessed March 1, 2022).

[32] See https://www.asco.org/news-initiatives/current-initiatives/cancer-care-initiatives/mcode-standard-data-ehr (accessed September 7, 2022).

[33] See https://www.ashresearchcollaborative.org/s/ (accessed September 7, 2022).

[34] See https://reaganudall.org/programs/research/real-world-data (accessed September 7, 2022).

[35] See https://friendsofcancerresearch.org/ (accessed September 7, 2022).

ONC: Advancing Interoperability and Innovation in Health IT

ONC is charged with advancing the development and uptake of an interoperable health IT infrastructure for the United States, said Avinash Shanbhag, executive director of the ONC Office of Technology. Under the Health Information Technology for Economic and Clinical Health (HITECH) Act,[36] ONC was specifically charged with certifying EHR systems to ensure they meet standards and support electronic HIE.[37] Currently, he said, 96 percent of hospitals and 90 percent of physicians providing care in the outpatient setting are using EHRs that are certified by ONC.

To promote interoperability of EHR systems, ONC established the United States Core Data for Interoperability (USCDI),[38] which Shanbhag said includes the data elements that are to be captured, stored, and exchanged by all ONC-certified EHR technologies.[39] The USCDI is updated annually based on agency and industry input so that the minimum data set grows to meet evolving needs. ONC has also established certification criteria for the EHR APIs developed to facilitate data exchange, and API Conditions of Maintenance and Certification, which apply to the third-party developers of certified EHR APIs. Another area of focus for ONC is interoperability of health information networks. Shanbhag described ONC's creation of a Trusted Exchange Framework Common Agreement, which establishes national standards and a governance process to enable data exchange among different networks.[40]

ONC is also working with other agencies to foster innovation in health IT. For example, Shanbhag said ONC is collaborating with the CDC to develop standards for the development of EHR-integrated clinical decision support technology.

CMS: Enabling EHRs to Better Support Health Care Data Exchange

Lara Strawbridge, director of the Division of Ambulatory Payment Models at the CMS Center for Medicare and Medicaid Innovation (CMMI), said the agency is working to facilitate better health care data exchange among payers, health care systems, clinical practices, and patients by leveraging sup-

---

[36] See https://www.healthit.gov/topic/laws-regulation-and-policy/health-it-legislation (accessed September 1, 2022).

[37] See https://www.healthit.gov/topic/certification-ehrs/certification-health-it (accessed May 18, 2022).

[38] See https://www.healthit.gov/isa/united-states-core-data-interoperability-uscdi (accessed September 1, 2022).

[39] See https://www.healthit.gov/isa/united-states-core-data-interoperability-uscdi (accessed May 18, 2022).

[40] See https://rce.sequoiaproject.org (accessed May 18, 2022).

port, incentives, and requirements. "Better health care data exchange ... will inform decision making for patients and their care providers, it will support and improve patient care and outcomes, and ideally, it will reduce the administrative burden on providers and payers," she said. For example, the Oncology Care Model[41] emphasizes improving patient–clinician communication through activities such as care planning. Although there have been implementation challenges (e.g., changing the practice culture, adapting workflows, modifying the EHR to capture the elements of the care plan), she said that practices participating in the model have shared anecdotally that implementing a care plan has improved their communication with patients. However, Strawbridge noted the lack of metrics for assessing how well these solutions improve communication.

In May 2020 the CMS Interoperability and Patient Access final rule[42] was published and requires certified EHRs to share data with patients, care providers, and payers via secure APIs, starting January 1, 2022. This rule both enables the sharing of health data between patient and clinician via the patient's personal health app and mandates that EHRs support data exchange among clinicians and with payers, Strawbridge explained. She added that CMS is planning to undertake rulemaking to address some of the specific operational challenges pertaining to payer-to-payer data exchange. Other CMS activities to promote interoperability include aligning with ONC's USCDI initiative (the standardized vocabulary for core data elements, previously discussed by Shanbhag) and studying how technology tools could be leveraged to streamline payer processes (e.g., prior authorization).

The CMS Quality Payment Program is shifting clinician payment from a fee-for-service model to one that rewards quality and value. The Merit-Based Incentive Payment System (MIPS) adjusts payment based on how clinicians score on quality- and cost-improving activities and on promoting interoperability. Strawbridge noted that the category on promoting interoperability performance requires clinicians to use certified EHR technology (CEHRT). She also discussed alternative payment models (APM), including a MIPS APM and an Advanced APM.[43] Use of CEHRT is an important element of the Quality Payment Program, and Strawbridge said that use of CEHRT is required for a clinician to be eligible for the highest scores in this program.

---

[41] See https://innovation.cms.gov/innovation-models/oncology-care (accessed September 1, 2022).

[42] See https://www.cms.gov/newsroom/fact-sheets/interoperability-and-patient-access-factsheet (accessed September 1, 2022).

[43] For more information about alternative payment models, see https://qpp.cms.gov/apms/overview#:~:text=An%20Advanced%20APM%20is%20a,reporting%20requirements%20and%20payment%20adjustment (accessed September 7, 2022).

The Oncology Care Model also requires the use of CEHRT as one of its six practice redesign activities, Strawbridge said. Further, CMMI considers using CEHRT to be "foundational" to successful implementation of the other practice redesign activities. Similarly, the Radiation Oncology Model, if implemented, would require use of CEHRT by participants in the Advanced APM, and Strawbridge said use of CEHRT is foundational to the other aspects of this model as well.[44]

CMMI published an informal Request for Information in late 2019, calling for input on a new oncology model that would require the use of CEHRT and potentially require "gradual implementation of electronic patient-reported outcomes." CMMI is also looking to refresh its strategy and "move toward a health system that achieves equitable outcomes through high-quality, affordable, person-centered care."[45] Strawbridge highlighted two pillars of this initiative. The "support innovation" pillar is focused on innovations that enable integrated person-centered care, including "actionable, practice-specific data and . . . technology." The "partner-to-achieve system transformation" pillar seeks to engage "payers, purchasers, providers, states, and beneficiaries to improve quality, achieve equitable outcomes, and reduce health care costs."

Addressing the Challenges of Integrating SDOH Data in the EHR

Robert Carlson, chief executive officer of the National Comprehensive Cancer Network, discussed the challenges clinicians face in documenting and using key SDOH data in a patient's EHR. Richardson said that SDOH data are not consistently captured in EHRs. She referred participants to a prior National Cancer Policy Forum workshop that examined SDOH in the context of cancer and discussed opportunities to capture SDOH data for patients with cancer.[46] Sim said that OSTP has recently formed an SDOH interagency policy committee to engage collaborators to understand end-user data needs. OSTP is interested in how data on SDOH are integrated, accessed, and used. Sim highlighted the importance of creating a collaborative EHR environment that facilitates access to SDOH data but also makes patients feel comfortable that their data are secure and are being used for their benefit. It is important to always be mindful that these data are not just numbers and information; they are connected to a person, she said. Shanbhag referred to the Gravity Project (mentioned in the section on Improving Data Collection and Display

---

[44] Strawbridge noted that Congress has prohibited implementation of the Radiation Oncology Model before January 1, 2023.

[45] See https://innovation.cms.gov/strategic-direction-whitepaper (accessed May 18, 2022).

[46] See https://nap.nationalacademies.org/catalog/25835/applying-big-data-to-address-the-social-determinants-of-health-in-oncology (accessed May 18, 2022).

to Support Clinical Decision Making), which he described as a "bottom-up approach" to develop standards for capturing SDOH data, and noted that ONC's July 2021 update to USCDI included SDOH-related data elements.

Coordinating EHR-Related Efforts across Federal Agencies and with Partners

Multiple federal agencies have interests in improving the functionality and usability of EHRs for cancer care, surveillance, and research, said Nicole Dowling, associate director for science in the CDC Division of Cancer Prevention and Control. She noted that many speakers highlighted the need to prioritize and improve coordination of efforts across agencies and with nonfederal partners. Sim observed that many of the challenges of coordinating agency efforts are not administration- or agency-specific. She reiterated that OSTP is well positioned to stimulate collaboration and coordination across the federal sector. OSTP is also interested in bringing federal sector partners together with state, local, tribal, and territorial authorities to coordinate public health infrastructure efforts. Sim added that coordinating efforts with academia and the private sector are also key to success. Shanbhag said that the annual update to USCDI is a transparent, collaborative process that is based on feedback collected from federal agencies, industry, and other key participants over the prior year.[47]

Carlson observed that the need for structured data, standardized formats, and interoperability standards seems to be broadly acknowledged, and he asked what role the federal government could take to promote the partnerships necessary to advance progress. Richardson suggested that coordination of federal agency efforts involves a "push–pull" strategy. Agencies are often required or compelled by ONC or Congress to coordinate efforts, but there is also a push from external parties for agencies to collaborate. She said that agencies need to look beyond their own data and programs and seek opportunities to work together. Penberthy agreed that many in the public health, informatics, and health system communities are interested in having EHRs with structured data, but challenges abound. For example, she said it "costs an inordinate amount of money for health care systems to install new EHRs." She acknowledged the efforts by CMS to achieve structured and consistent billing across all insurers (government and commercial) and suggested there could be an opportunity for CMS to press commercial EHR vendors to develop structured formats for public health reporting and data exchange. A challenge, however, would be the wide variability across vendors and products.

---

[47] See https://www.healthit.gov/isa/ONDEC (accessed May 18, 2022).

Kluetz highlighted the importance of intergovernmental discussion to identify what information different end users need from the EHR and of engaging the key partners in driving the standards. For example, if one seeks to efficiently gather substantial evidence of treatment efficacy from the EHR, the FDA should be part of the conversation about data needs when standardized data formats are being developed and implemented by ONC or CMMI.

REFLECTIONS

Levy shared closing reflections on the themes that emerged from the workshop discussions. She said it was clear from the presentations and discussions that "EHRs are evolving and will continue to evolve." The EHR is "a living thing" that needs to adapt to meet new priorities and overcome new challenges. For example, there was discussion throughout the workshop about the need to work in partnership with patients and the need for EHR data to be accessible for research and to support a continuously learning health care system.

Recurrent themes of discussion included:

- **Interoperability** There has been significant progress toward interoperability *within* EHR networks that is contributing to better patient management, Levy said, but interoperability also needs to enable integration of information across EHR systems from different vendors. There was discussion of emerging standards and incentives that are driving interoperability forward. Several speakers also suggested revisiting the HIPAA Privacy Rule to facilitate the sharing of EHR data.
- **Structured data standards** Although there has been progress in developing structured data standards in oncology, incentives for implementation are lacking. Levy said that a "national will" is needed to drive the uptake of structured data standards that can enable the ability to enter data once and use it for multiple purposes.
- **Clinical decision support** Locally configured oncology clinical decision support tools are being implemented in EHRs, and there were examples of how they can be updated rapidly when needed (e.g., to address a medication shortage). Some of the EHR-embedded clinical decision support tools for oncology that were discussed included screening guidelines, treatment pathways, chemotherapy order sets, and ePROs. However, the ability to share knowledge, best practices, and validated EHR clinical decision support tools across vendors and health systems is lacking, Levy said. Further, the user experience when interfacing with new decision support tools that have been integrated into an existing EHR system is often less than ideal.

- **Balancing EHR innovation with careforce burnout** Throughout the workshop the point was made that innovation in EHRs for oncology care, research, and surveillance need to consider the clinical workflow, so that it does not further increase the documentation and cognitive burden on oncology clinicians.

Levy pointed out that the critical challenges and opportunities being discussed today are different from those of five years ago, and there will be new challenges and opportunities five years from now.

REFERENCES

Albers, D. J., M. Levine, B. Gluckman, H. Ginsberg, G. Hripcsak, and L. Mamykina. 2017. Personalized glucose forecasting for type 2 diabetes using data assimilation. *PLOS Computational Biology* 13(4):e1005232. https://doi.org/10.1371/journal.pcbi.1005232.

Alkureishi, M. A., T. Johnson, J. Nichols, M. Dhodapkar, M. K. Czerwiec, K. Wroblewski, V. M. Arora, and W. W. Lee. 2021. Impact of an educational comic to enhance patient–physician–electronic health record engagement: Prospective observational study. *JMIR Human Factors* 8(2):e25054. https://doi.org/10.2196/25054.

Basch, E. 2010. The missing voice of patients in drug-safety reporting. *The New England Journal of Medicine* 362(10):865–869.

Basch, E., A. M. Deal, A. C. Dueck, H. I. Scher, M. G. Kris, C. Hudis, and D. Schrag. 2017. Overall survival results of a trial assessing patient-reported outcomes for symptom monitoring during routine cancer treatment. *JAMA* 318(2):197–198.

Basch, E., D. Schrag, S. Henson, J. Jansen, B. Ginos, A.M. Stover, P. Carr, P.A. Spears, M. Jonsson, A. M. Deal, A. V. Bennett, G. Thanarajasingam, L. J. Rogak, B. B. Reeve, C. Snyder, D. Bruner, D. Cella, L. A. Kottschade, J. Perlmutter, C. Geoghegan, C. A. Samuel-Ryals, B. Given, G. L. Mazza, R. Miller, J. F. Strasser, D. M. Zylla, A. Weiss, V. S. Blinder, and A. C. Dueck. 2022. Effect of electronic symptom monitoring on patient-reported outcomes among patients with metastatic cancer: A randomized clinical trial. *JAMA* 327(24):2413–2422.

Benard, V. B., J. E. Jackson, A. Greek, V. Senkomago, W. K. Huh, C. C. Thomas, and L. C. Richardson. 2021. A population study of screening history and diagnostic outcomes of women with invasive cervical cancer. *Cancer Medicine* 10(12):4127–4137. https://doi.org/10.1002/cam4.3951.

Bernstam, E. V., J. L, Warner, J. C. Krauss, E. Ambinder, W. S. Rubinstein, G. Komatsoulis, R. S. Miller, and J. L. Chen. 2022. Quantitating and assessing interoperability between electronic health records. *Journal of the American Medical Informatics Association*. 29(5):753–760. https://doi.org/10.1093/jamia/ocab289.

Carayon, P., and M. E. Salwei. 2021. Moving toward a sociotechnical systems approach to continuous health information technology design: The path forward for improving electronic health record usability and reducing clinician burnout. *Journal of the American Medical Informatics Association* 28(5):1026–1028. https://doi.org/10.1093/jamia/ocab002.

Carayon, P., A. Wooldridge, P. Hoonakker, A. S. Hundtand, and M. M. Kelly. 2020. SEIPS 3.0: Human-centered design of the patient journey for patient safety. *Applied Ergonomics* 84:103303. https://doi.org/10.1016/j.apergo.2019.103033.

Cusack, C. M., G. Hripcsak, M. Bloomrosen, S. T. Rosenbloom, C. A. Weaver, A. Wright, D. K. Vawdrey, J. Walker, and L. Mamykina. 2013. The future state of clinical data capture and documentation: A report from AMIA's 2011 Policy Meeting. *Journal of the American Medical Informatics Association* 20(1):134–140. https://doi.org/10.1136/amiajnl-2012-001093.

Denis, F., E. Basch, A. L. Septans, J. Bennouna, T. Urban, A. C. Dueck, and C. Letellier. 2019. Two-year survival comparing web-based symptom monitoring vs routine surveillance following treatment for lung cancer. *JAMA* 321(3):306–307.

Finkelstein, J., M. R. Cabrera, and G. Hripcsak. 2000. Internet-based home asthma telemonitoring: Can patients handle the technology? *Chest* 117(1):148–155.

Gajra, A., B. Bapat, Y. Jeune-Smith, C. Nabhan, A. J. Klink, D. Liassou, S. Mehta, and B. Feinberg. 2020. Frequency and causes of burnout in U.S. community oncologists in the era of electronic health records. *JCO Oncology Practice* 16(4):e357–e365.

Gawande, A. "The bell curve." *The New Yorker* December 6, 2004.

Gawande, A. "Why doctors hate their computers." *The New Yorker* November 12, 2018.

Gombar, S., A. Callahan, R. Califf, R. Harrington, and N. H. Shah. 2019. It is time to learn from patients like mine. *NPJ Digital Medicine* 2(16). https://doi.org/10.1038/s41746-019-0091-3.

Haider, A., K. Tanco, M. Epner, A. Azhar, J. Williams, D. D. Liu, and E. Bruera. 2018. Physicians' compassion, communication skills, and professionalism with and without physicians' use of an examination room computer: A randomized clinical trial. *JAMA Oncology* 4(6):879–881. https://doi.org/10.1001/jamaoncol.2018.0343.

Hayes, G., G. Abowd, J. Davis, M. Blount, M. Ebling, and E. D. Mynatt. 2008. "Opportunities for pervasive computing in chronic cancer care." In *Proceedings of the 6th International Conference on Pervasive Computing* (Berlin, Heidelberg: Springer-Verlag), 262–279.

Himmelstein, G., D. Bates, and L. Zhou. 2022. Examination of stigmatizing language in the electronic health record. *JAMA Network Open* 5(1):e2144967. https://doi.org/10.1001/jamanetworkopen.2021.44967.

Hirsch, J. S., J. S. Tanenbaum, S. Lipsky Gorman, C. Liu, E. Schmitz, D. Hashorva, A. Ervits, D. Vawdrey, M. Sturm, and N. Elhadad. 2015. HARVEST, a longitudinal patient record summarizer. *Journal of the American Medical Informatics Association* 22(2):263–274.

Hughes-Halbert, C., M. Jefferson, C. G. Allen, O. A. Babatunde, R. Drake, P. Angel, S. J. Savage, L, Frey, M. Lilly, T. Obi, and J. Obeid. 2021. Racial differences in patient portal activation and research enrollment among patients with prostate cancer. *JCO Clinical Cancer Informatics* 5:768–774. https://doi.org/10.1200/CCI.20.00131.

IOM (Institute of Medicine). 2000. *To err is human: Building a safer health system*. Washington, DC: The National Academies Press.

IOM. 2009. *Beyond the HIPAA Privacy Rule: Enhancing privacy, improving health through research*. Washington, DC: The National Academies Press.

Jacobs, M., J. Clawson, and E. D. Mynatt. 2014. Cancer navigation: Opportunities and challenges for facilitating the breast cancer journey. In *CSCW 2014—Proceedings of the 17th ACM Conference on Computer Supported Cooperative Work and Social Computing* (Association for Computing Machinery), 1467–1478.

Jacobs, M., J. Hopkins, M. Mumber, and E. Mynatt. 2019. Usability evaluation of an adaptive information recommendation system for breast cancer patients. *AMIA Annual Symposium Proceedings* 2019:494–503.

Jacobs, M., J. Johnson, and E. D. Mynatt. 2018. MyPath: Investigating breast cancer patients' use of personalized health information. *Proceedings of the ACM on Human–Computer Interaction* 2(CSCW): Article 78, 1–21.

Jacobs, M. L., J. Clawson, and E. D. Mynatt. 2017. Articulating a patient-centered design space for cancer journeys. *EAI Endorsed Transactions on Pervasive Health and Technology* 3(9):e5. https://doi.org/10.4108/eai.21-3-2017.152394.

Kortum, P. T. 2016. *Usability assessment: How to measure the usability of products, services, and systems*. Santa Monica, CA: The Human Factors and Ergonomics Society.

Lafferty, M., M. Manojlovich, J. J. Griggs, N. Wright, M. Harrod, and C. R. Friese. 2021. Clinicians report barriers and facilitators to high-quality ambulatory oncology care. *Cancer Nursing* 44(5):E303–E310. https://doi.org/10.1097/ncc.0000000000000832.

Lichtner, V., B. D. Franklin, L. Dalla-Pozza, and J. I. Westbrook. 2020. Electronic ordering and the management of treatment interdependencies: A qualitative study of paediatric chemotherapy. *BMC Medical Informatics and Decision Making* 20(1):193. https://doi.org/10.1186/s12911-020-01212-z.

Lichtner, V., and M. Baysari. 2021. Electronic display of a patient treatment over time: A perspective on clinicians' burn-out. *BMJ Health & Care Informatics* 28(1):e100281.

Mamykina, L., E. M. Heitkemper, A. M. Smaldone, R. Kukafka, H. J. Cole-Lewis, P. G. Davidson, E. D. Mynatt, A. Cassells, J. N. Tobin, and G. Hripcsak. 2017. Personal discovery in diabetes self-management: Discovering cause and effect using self-monitoring data. *Journal of Biomedical Informatics* 76:1–8. https://doi.org/10.1016/j.jbi.2017.09.013.

Mamykina, L., E. M. Heitkemper, A. M. Smaldone, R. Kukafka, H. Cole-Lewis, P. G. Davidson, E. D. Mynatt, J. N. Tobin, A. Cassells, C. Goodman, and G. Hripcsak. 2016. Structured scaffolding for reflection and problem solving in diabetes self-management: Qualitative study of mobile diabetes detective. *Journal of the American Medical Informatics Association* 23(1):129–136.

McCleary, N. J., M. J. Healey, S. Weng, A. B. Song, R. I. Lederman, H. Z. Ramelson, A. J. Wagner, and G. A. Abel. 2018. Perceptions of oncologists about sharing clinic notes with patients. *Oncologist* 24(1):e46–e48.

Melnick, E. R., A. Fong, B. Nath, B. Williams, R. M. Ratwani, R. Goldstein, R. T. O'Connell, C. A. Sinsky, D. Marchalik, and M. Mete. 2021. Analysis of electronic health record use and clinical productivity and their association with physician turnover. *JAMA Network Open* 4(10):e2128790.

Moll, J., and Å. Cajander. 2020. Oncology health-care professionals' perceived effects of patient accessible electronic health records 6 years after launch: A survey study at a major university hospital in Sweden. *Health Informatics Journal* 26(2):1392–1403.

NASEM (National Academies of Sciences, Engineering, and Medicine). 2019. *Developing and sustaining an effective and resilient oncology careforce: Proceedings of a workshop*. Washington, DC: The National Academies Press.

Patel, M. S., S. C. Day, S. D. Halpern, C. W. Hanson, J. R. Martinez, S. Honeywell, Jr., and K. G. Volpp. 2016. Generic medication prescription rates after health system-wide redesign of default options within the electronic health record. *JAMA Internal Medicine* 176(6):847–848. doi:10.1001/jamainternmed.2016.1691.

Patt, D., L. Wilfong, K. E. Hudson, A. Patel, H. Books, B. Pearson, R. Boren, S. Patil, K. Olson-Celli, and E. Basch. 2021. Implementation of electronic patient-reported outcomes for symptom monitoring in a large multisite community oncology practice: Dancing the Texas two-step through a pandemic. *JCO Clinical Cancer Informatics* 5:615-621.

Pickering, B. W., V. Herasevich, A. Ahmed, and O. Gajic. 2010. Novel representation of clinical information in the ICU: Developing user interfaces which reduce information overload. *Applied Clinical Informatics* 1(2):116–131. https://doi.org/10.4338/aci-2009-12-cr-0027.

Prey, J. E., F. Polubriaginof, L. V. Grossman, R. Masterson Creber, D. Tsapepas, R. Perotte, M. Qian, S. Restaino, S. Bakken, G. Hripcsak, L. Efird, J. Underwood, and D. K. Vawdrey. 2018. Engaging hospital patients in the medication reconciliation process using tablet computers. *Journal of the American Medical Informatics Association* 25(11):1460–1469.

Rousek, J. B., and M. S. Hallbeck. 2011. Improving medication management through the redesign of the hospital code cart medication drawer. *Human Factors* 53(6):626–636. https://doi.org/10.1177/0018720811426427.

Shaverdian, N., E. M. Chang, F. I. Chu, E. G. Morasso, M. A. Pfeffer, E. M. Cheng, A. Wu, S. A. McCloskey, A. C. Raldow, and M. L. Steinberg. 2019. Impact of open access to physician notes on radiation oncology patients: Results from an exploratory survey. *Practical Radiation Oncology* 9(2):102–107. https://doi.org/10.1016/j.prro.2018.10.004.

Shulman, L. N., L. K. Sheldon, and E. J. Benz. 2020. The future of cancer care in the United States—overcoming workforce capacity limitations. *JAMA Oncology* 6(3):327–328.

Steitz, B. D., and M. A. Levy. 2017. A social network analysis of cancer provider collaboration. *AMIA Annual Symposium Proceedings* 2016:1987–1996.

Takvorian, S. U., J. Bekelman, R. S. Beidas, R. Schnoll, A. B. W. Clifton, T. Salam, P. Gabriel, E. P. Wileyto, C. A. Scott, D. A. Asch, A. M. Buttenheim, K. A. Rendle, K. Chaiyachati, R. C. Shelton, S. Ware, C. Chivers, L. M. Schuchter, P. Kumar, L. N. Shulman, N. O'Connor, A. Lieberman, K. Zentgraf, and R. B. Parikh. 2021. Behavioral economic implementation strategies to improve serious illness communication between clinicians and high-risk patients with cancer: Protocol for a cluster randomized pragmatic trial. *Implementation Science* 16, 90. https://doi.org/10.1186/s13012-021-01156-6.

Takvorian, S. U., V. P. Ladage, E. P. Wileyto, D. S. Mace, R. S. Beidas, L. N. Shulman, and J. E. Bekelman. 2020. Association of behavioral nudges with high-value evidence-based prescribing in oncology. *JAMA Oncology* 6(7):1104–1106.

Tempero, M. 2021. Open Notes are here: Are we ready? *Journal of the National Comprehensive Cancer Network* 19(5):477.

Tetzlaff, E. D., H. M. Hylton, K. J. Ruth, Z. Hasse, and M. J. Hall. 2022. Changes in burnout among oncology physician assistants between 2015 and 2019. *JCO Oncology Practice* 18(1):e47–e59.

Thaler, R. H., and C. Sunstein. 2009. *Nudge: Improving decisions about health, wealth, and happiness.* New York: Penguin Books.

Waddell, K. J., P. D. Shah, S. Adusumalli, and M. S. Patel. 2020. Using behavioral economics and technology to improve outcomes in cardio-oncology. *JACC CardioOncology* 2(1):84–96. https://doi.org/10.1016/j.jaccao.2020.02.006

Zhu, V. J., A. Lenert, B. E. Bunnell, J. S. Obeid, M. Jefferson, and C. H. Halbert. 2019. Automatically identifying social isolation from clinical narratives for patients with prostate cancer. *BMC Medical Informatics Decision Making* 19(1):43. https://doi.org/10.1186/s12911-019-0795-y.

Appendix A

Statement of Task

A planning committee of the National Academies of Sciences, Engineering, and Medicine will plan and host a 1.5-day public workshop that will examine opportunities to improve patient care and outcomes through collaborations to enhance innovation in the development, implementation, and use of electronic health records (EHRs) in oncology care, research, and surveillance. The workshop will feature invited presentations and panel discussions on topics that may include:

- Challenges and opportunities to optimize the functionality and usability of EHRs in oncology care, such as efforts to standardize essential data, data presentation, and decision support, as well as the need to address governance structures and processes to prioritize and implement these improvements.
- Standardization of oncology EHR documentation to facilitate care and communication among clinicians and patients.
- Capture of data on social determinants of health.
- Opportunities to collect and integrate patient reported outcomes measures into EHRs and produce real-time or more timely data to guide cancer care and facilitate cancer research and surveillance.
- Ongoing initiatives to enhance EHR structure, data standardization, and interoperability with the goal of improving care and real-world clinical data collection for research, surveillance, and improvement of care quality. This may include essential data to be collected, and methods for doing so, as well as integration of genomics data.

- Use of computing technologies such as artificial intelligence to enhance EHRs and facilitate the use of EHRs to improve clinical care and enhance oncology research.
- Opportunities to better align incentives to ensure that EHRs offered by vendors meet the needs of the various users in oncology (e.g., patients, clinicians, payers, researchers).
- Past and ongoing examples of collaborations to conceptualize and implement innovations in EHRs for cancer care, research, and surveillance.
- Policies to foster redesign of EHRs to serve as a functional component of surveillance systems to advance oncology care.

The planning committee will develop the agenda for the workshop sessions, select and invite speakers and discussants, and moderate the discussions. A proceedings of the presentations and discussions at the workshop will be prepared by a designated rapporteur in accordance with institutional guidelines.

Appendix B

Workshop Agenda

FEBRUARY 28, 2022

9:30 a.m. **Welcome from the National Cancer Policy Forum**
Planning Committee Co-Chairs:
- Mia Levy, Foundation Medicine, Inc.
- Lawrence N. Shulman, University of Pennsylvania Abramson Cancer Center

9:40 a.m. **Session 1: Overview of the Use of EHRs in Oncology Care, Research, and Surveillance**
Co-moderators:
- Mia Levy, Foundation Medicine, Inc.
- Lawrence N. Shulman, University of Pennsylvania Abramson Cancer Center

Session Objective: To review the current state and trends of EHRs and discuss the evidence base for the design, development, and use of EHRs in cancer care, research, and surveillance.

Technical and Contextual Evolution of EHRs
Mia Levy, Foundation Medicine, Inc.

The Electronic Health Record: From the View of the Oncologist
Lawrence N. Shulman, University of Pennsylvania Abramson Cancer Center

Facilitator of Trust or Mediator of Communication: The EHR and the Patient–Physician Relationship
Gwen Darien, National Patient Advocate Foundation

Integrating Social Determinants of Health in EHRs: Ethical and Social Justice Issues
Chanita Hughes-Halbert, USC Norris Comprehensive Cancer Center

Quality Improvement and Research Perspective
Neal J. Meropol, Flatiron Health

Panel Discussion with Speakers

11:10 a.m. Break

11:20 a.m. **Session 2: Opportunities to Improve the Patient-Facing Aspects of EHRs**
Co-moderators:
- Etta D. Pisano, Harvard Medical School/American College of Radiology
- Robin Yabroff, American Cancer Society

Session Objective: To explore opportunities and approaches to improve the patient-facing aspects of EHRs to empower patients and improve patient care and outcomes.

The Impact of EHRs on the Physician–Patient Relationship
Jyoti D. Patel, Northwestern University

Integrating Patient-Reported Outcomes into Electronic Health Record Systems in Oncology
Ethan Basch, University of North Carolina at Chapel Hill

Today's Patient Portal and Sharing of Patient Data across EHR Systems for Cancer Care and Research
Travis J. Osterman, Vanderbilt University Medical Center

Using the EHR to "Nudge" Evidence-Based Cancer Care
Samuel U. Takvorian, Penn Medicine

Next-Generation EHRs to Facilitate Oncology Care
George Hripcsak, Columbia University

Panel Discussion with Speakers

12:50 p.m.   **Lunch Break**

1:50 p.m.   **Session 3: Opportunities to Optimize the Functionality and Usability of EHRs in Oncology Care**
Co-moderators:
- Bradley Malin, Vanderbilt University Medical Center
- Alexander Melamed, Columbia University Medical Center

Session Objective: To examine the challenges and opportunities to optimize the functionality and usability of EHRs in clinical workflow to meet the needs of the various users in oncology care.

Oncology Care Pathways: Importance and Relation to Current EHRs' Functionality and Opportunities for Improvement
Robin Zon, Michiana Hematology Oncology

Opportunities for Decision Support through the Use of EHRs
Mary M. Ichiuji, Kaiser Permanente

Efficiency of EHR Use and Management in Creating an Ideal Workspace and Presentation of Critical Data for Oncology-Specific Care Providers
Shilo Anders, Vanderbilt University

Interface between Electronic Systems and Humans: View from Outside of Medicine
Elizabeth Mynatt, Northeastern University

Human Factors Engineering for EHR Design in Oncology Care: The Patient Experience across the Cancer Care Continuum
Pascale Carayon, University of Wisconsin-Madison

An Industry Perspective
Jenna Date, Allscripts Hospital and Health Systems

Panel Discussion with Speakers

3:25 p.m.   **Break**

3:35 p.m.   **Session 4: Roundtable—Innovative Strategies to Improve EHR Data Collection to Support Care Quality and Research Initiatives**
Co-moderators:
- Neal J. Meropol, Flatiron Health
- Lara Strawbridge, Center for Medicare and Medicaid Innovation, Centers for Medicare & Medicaid Services

Session Objective: To discuss new approaches and opportunities to enhance EHR structure, data collection and standardization, interoperability, and EHR integration to improve clinical care and enhance oncology research.

Clinician Perspective
Tufia C. Haddad, Mayo Clinic College of Medicine and Sciences

Opportunities and Challenges: Entry of Critical Structured Data into EHRs
Monica Bertagnolli, Brigham and Women's Hospital and Dana-Farber Cancer Institute

Researcher Perspective: Opportunities for Improved Research
Jeremy L. Warner, Vanderbilt University

Quality Improvement Initiatives: Opportunities for Improved Quality of Care
Barry Russo, The Center for Cancer and Blood Disorders

Payer Perspective
Reed V. Tuckson, Black Coalition Against COVID and Tuckson Health Connections, LLC

Panel Discussion with Panelists

APPENDIX B

4:50 p.m.   **Closing Remarks**

5:00 p.m.   **Adjourn**

MARCH 1, 2022

9:00 a.m.   **Welcome and Overview of Day 2**
Planning Committee Co-Chairs
- Mia Levy, Foundation Medicine, Inc.
- Lawrence N. Shulman, University of Pennsylvania Abramson Cancer Center

9:05 a.m.   **Session 5: The Roles of Federal Agencies to Advance Progress in EHRs**
Co-moderators:
- Robert W. Carlson, National Comprehensive Cancer Network
- Nicole F. Dowling, Centers for Disease Control and Prevention

Session Objective: To explore current collaborations and initiatives to conceptualize and implement innovations in EHRs and discuss potential policy incentives for the adoption of improved EHRs in cancer care, research, and surveillance.

Potential Role of Science and Technology Policy in Advancement of EHRs
Bich-Thuy (Twee) Sim, Office of Science and Technology Policy and the Department of Defense

Advancing Progress in EHRs: Cancer Surveillance as an Example
Lynne Penberthy, National Cancer Institute

Electronic Health Records for Public Health Planning and Research
Lisa C. Richardson, Centers for Disease Control and Prevention

Leveraging Electronic Health Records: Expanding Opportunities for Evidence Generation
Paul G. Kluetz, Oncology Center of Excellence, Food and Drug Administration

Ready, Set, Go!: Leveraging EHRs for Innovation
Avinash Shanbhag, Office of Technology, Office of the National Coordinator

CMMI Perspective
Lara Strawbridge, Center for Medicare and Medicaid Innovation, Centers for Medicare & Medicaid Services

Panel Discussion with Speakers

10:35 a.m.   **Break**

10:45 a.m.   **Session 6: Policies to Foster EHR Redesign to Advance Progress in Cancer Care, Research, and Surveillance**
Co-moderators:
- Mimi Huizinga, ImmunoGen, Inc.
- Robert A. Winn, Virginia Commonwealth University Massey Cancer Center

Session Objective: To discuss potential policy levers and actionable strategies to enhance innovation in the development, implementation, and use of EHRs in oncology care, research, and surveillance.

Panelists (Session Co-moderators)
- Representing Session 1: Lawrence Shulman
- Representing Session 2: Etta Pisano
- Representing Session 3: Bradley Malin
- Representing Session 4: Lara Strawbridge
- Representing Session 5: Nicole Dowling

Open Discussion

11:50 a.m.   **Closing Remarks**
Mia Levy, Foundation Medicine, Inc.
Planning Committee Co-Chair

12:00 p.m.   **Adjourn**